Latina Facial Skincare

Beautiful and Healthy Skin Guide:
Practical Tips and Advice
Catalina Charpentier B.

ISBN: 978-1-961176-03-4 (eBook)

ISBN: 978-1-961176-04-1 (Paperback)

ISBN: 978-1-961176-05-8 (Hardback)

Publisher: ARTEMIX BEAUTY, Owasso, Oklahoma
Website: www.artemixbeauty.com
Instagram: @artemixbeauty
Facebook: @artemixbeauty

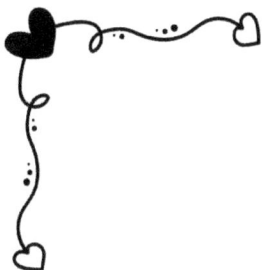

JUST FOR YOU

NATURAL EXTRACTS TO ENHANCE YOUR COSMETICS

Basic DIY Anti-Aging Secrets using Plant-Based Ingredients

CATALIANA CHARPENTIER B.

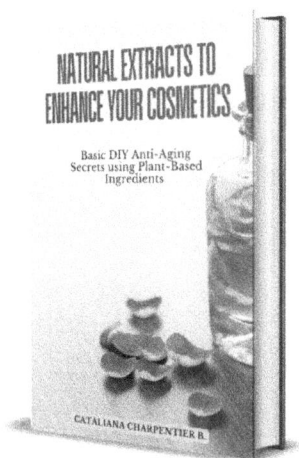

A FREE GIVEAWAY

Learn about Natural Anti-Aging Extracts

www.artemixbeauty.com

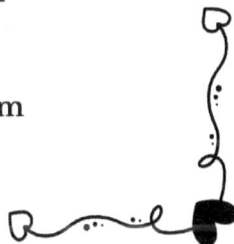

Gift

www.artemixbeauty.com

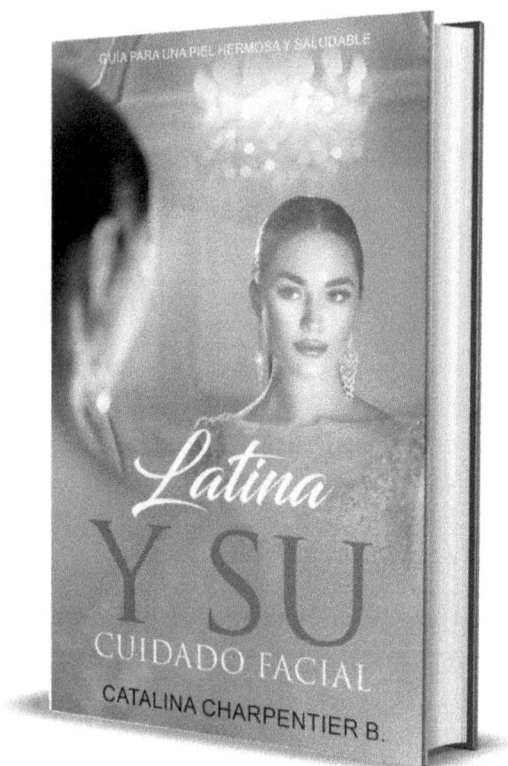

GUÍA PARA UNA PIEL HERMOSA Y SALUDABLE

Latina

Y SU

CUIDADO FACIAL

CATALINA CHARPENTIER B.

Descubre los secretos para lucir
espectacular en cada página.
Aprende sobre el cuidado de la
piel, la elección de productos y
los mejores suplementos para
rejuvenecer tu rostro.

Contents

Introduction

The skin of us Latina women, unlike a very white skin, does not develop expression lines easily. That being said, it is relatively simple to calculate the biological age of our skin by its quality, the presence of spots, the appearance of the eye contour and loss of volume on the face.

The expression "That person does not age because she made a pact with the devil" was very familiar during my younger years. Throughout those years, I understood that maintaining a young skin does not depend on age or demonic pacts. It depends on knowing how to correctly identify your skin tone and type and acquiring appropriate skin care habits according to your specific needs.

First, it's important that you need to keep in mind that skincare is a journey, not the destination that becomes a chore on your to-do list. Think about it! In a few years, your skin will show how it was treated today. Good skin care is a journey to conscientiousness and the secret behind an ageless complexion.

Great first impressions start with having a healthy face, especially within our culture. The face is the first thing that people notice when interacting with you. What our skin reveals can have a positive impact on our relationships, but this does not mean that we should leave aside our values and personality. Having a healthy face is an ally that can help strengthen your confidence.

In these pages you will discover information based on my experience as a Dermacosmiatra and researcher. I will give you the necessary tools to achieve healthy skin and declare war on acne, spots, dark circles, dermatitis, scars, photoaging and other blemishes. In the same vein, I will provide you with effective solutions for our Latin skin type, with lots of valuable information about care and maintenance protocols according to your skin type and criteria for selecting skin-loving products. I will even share a guide to the best supplements that will complement the care and rejuvenation of your face. I will tell you everything!

It's never too late to start taking care of your skin the right way. I remember turning 35 when I noticed that the skin on my face had changed. My face no longer had a uniform color or the glow of hydrated skin. The dark spots and loss of volume around my eyes gave my face a much older look. My frown lines were prominently highlighted when I went out in the sun or laughed. My search began to uncover how to take care of my delicate skin and reverse all the damage.

The aging of our face is inevitable, however, I discovered that there are several things we can do to improve and slow down the aging process to look younger and feel great. This newfound knowledge motivated me to train professionally in dermocosmiatry. Dermocosmiatricians have many skills and can identify and treat certain lesions, deep clean the skin, and rejuvenate the face.

Gradually this purpose born of a personal need became a passion. As I acquired knowledge about skincare and facial rejuvenation, I discovered an incredible world around the operation of cosmetic chemistry on our skin, the good habits of its care, and the development of hypoallergenic formulas and products for use in professional aesthetics—an experience that helped me to found Bie Sante Aesthetic Center in Ecuador with its own cosmetic line of more than 25 products formulated in the market.

Currently, it is very easy to find extensive information and commercial recommendations related to skincare and the use of products. Many information sources, whether they be formal or informal, can be confusing if you are not a trained professional. One of the most common mistakes women make is to select a skincare regimen that is not suitable for their skin type, inadvertently causing more damage and resulting in a loss of time and money. There are a lot of half-truths and misinformation when it comes to skincare, one of them being that we don't need sunscreen during the winter. This myth holds that during winter, the sun is less likely to cause sunburn, therefore you don't need sunscreen. The thing is, skin-damaging ultraviolet rays are always present. If you are outside long enough during the winter you'll get sunburned, and neglecting the sunscreen will promote the development of wrinkles. We should keep in mind that everyone has different skin. Apart from ethnic group characteristics, genetics and lifestyle have a big influence on the overall condition of your skin. While there is a lot of information out there, most of it is relegated to the annals of troubleshooting.

Faced with the growing need for reliable skincare information, Artemix Beauty was born in the USA with the mission to provide you with the necessary tools to properly care for your skin. Skin of Latin origin has certain strengths and weaknesses, and we have specialized in the development and research of products and services for Latin skin. Through individualized skincare programs, the democratization of knowledge, and books filled with practical information, we want to empower you to put your best face forward. Journey with me as we discover the secrets to maintaining your beautiful skin simply and practically.

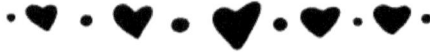

· ♥ · ♥ · ♥ · ♥ · ♥ ·

One

Latin Skin Tones

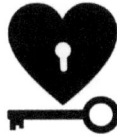

S kin care requires a bit more finesse than slapping on some moisturizer and hoping for the best. A good skincare routine helps to
keep the skin beautiful and nourished for years to come. In a market
flooded with care products, it can be incredibly difficult to select the
right skin care regimen for your skin type. Using the wrong products
can give the skin a dry, flaky, and dull appearance, or even trigger the
development of rashes and acne. Having a better understanding of
the evolution of skin color is a crucial first step in selecting suitable
products for your skin.

Mainstream thinking in research indicates a major change to early
human physiology around two million years ago. Early man ventured
from the forests and onto the East African savanna, where they had
to cope with increased sun exposure. Early humans developed more
sweat glands, and through millennia of natural selection, the human
body evolved so that each human now possesses roughly two million
sweat glands spread all over the body (Kirchweger, 2001). The increased sweat production helped our ancestors cope with the harsh

African sun better, with one caveat. Hairless skin dries out quicker and is vulnerable to damage, especially from sunlight.

Researchers have long assumed that melanin, which gives our skin color, absorbs ultraviolet light. But why does melanin absorb ultraviolet light? It turns out ultraviolet light has a detrimental effect on folate, otherwise known as folic acid or Vitamin B9. Folate plays a crucial role during pregnancy in embryonic development. An hour of exposure to intense sunlight is enough to significantly reduce folate levels in fair-skinned individuals (Jablonski, 1999), which can lead to abnormal fetal development.

Biochemist W. Farnsworth Loomis suggested that skin color and the need for vitamin D are linked. Loomis suggested that people living in the north, where daylight is weak, evolved fair skin to better aid the production of vitamin D, while people in the tropics evolved darker skin tones to prevent overproduction of the vitamin (Loomis, 1967).

If we look at the findings thus far it points to one thing—protection. Until the 1980s researchers could only guess how much ultraviolet radiation really reached Earth, but NASA helped to turn things around. In the late 70s, the space agency launched the Total Ozone Mapping Spectrometer to determine how much solar radiation reached Earth. The results gave researchers new insight into the mystery of skin color. Researchers found that skin color is an adaptation to higher levels of ultraviolet exposure (Jablonski & Chaplin, 2013). It turns out that people who live in the tropics have developed a darker skin tone to protect their body's folate reserves, while people who live far north developed fair skin to drink in sunlight for vitamin D production. The human body is fascinating indeed!

• ♥ • ♥ • ♥ • ♥ • ♥ •

Understanding Your Skin Tone

As Latinas, our skin is quite special. We tan easily and wrinkles take longer to appear on us when compared to our fair-skinned counterparts. This is all thanks to higher levels of melanin. Harvard professor and dermatologist, Dr. Thomas Fitzpatrick recognized that the skin's tanning ability significantly differed among individuals. The skin was consequently classified into six phototypes and the Fitzpatrick Scale was born. I'll explain the different skin types below.

- **Type I**

Albinism is often associated with this type. Individuals with Type I skin are beautifully pale, but can burn very easily in the sun. Type I skin can not tan and people with this type of skin should use sunscreen with a sun protection factor (SPF) of 75 and higher. Norse and Celtic peoples most commonly have this skin type. Quite commonly red or blonde hair with blue eyes and freckles complete the striking features.

- **Type II**

Commonly referred to as "Caucasian," this skin type is fairly light in color. Individuals with Type II skin typically have blonde hair and blue, green, or hazel eyes. They burn easily in the sun, but can tan, albeit very slowly. The tan is hard to notice in most cases, though!

Individuals with this skin type need to use sunscreen with an SPF of 50 and higher.

- **Type III**

Hailing from central European races, this skin type can range from luscious olive tones to lighter, yellowish tones. Individuals with this skin type typically have light brown hair with green or brown eyes. During winter, Type III skin tends to adopt a lighter tone, but can easily tan with some sun exposure. These skin types only need moderate protection from the sun and in most cases, an SPF of 35 to 50 will suffice.

- **Type IV**

This skin type is linked to the Mediterranean and American races. People with Type IV skin usually have light brown skin with brown hair and brown eyes. This skin type is quite resilient against sunburn and adopts delightful golden shades with ease. You'll only need an SPF of 15 to 35 to protect Type IV skin from the sun.

- **Type V**

Linked to Middle Eastern, Asian, and Latino races, this skin type can range from dark brown to a sultry caramel hue. Quick to tan and rarely prone to sunburn, you'll only need an SPF 15 for protection.

- **Type VI**

Linked to Afro-American and African races, this skin type has a multitude of delectable dark tones. Skin tones range from dark brown to black and are accompanied by sultry dark eyes and hair. This skin type is the most resistant against sunburn and tans with only a lick of sunlight.

Classifying Latina Skin

Latina skin is beautifully diverse, ranging from III, IV, and V on the Fitzpatrick scale. Latina skin is truly ageless! Gorgeous mocha, delectable bronzes, subtle honey, and many shades in-between define the very beauty of Latin skin. I'll share a few more reasons why you should love the skin you're in:

We don't develop expression lines easily. This is especially the case for medium to dark skin tones. That's because there is minimal muscle movement around the eyes, between the eyebrows, and on the forehead ("Self-Reported Facial Characteristics Associated with Aging in a Diverse Sample of Men and Women from a Multinational Web-Based Panel Survey," 2015). Less muscle movement minimizes wrinkling. This seems to be a shared characteristic among darker-skinned people, as studies have found that African American women share this interesting trait.

Better sun protection. Latinas with darker skin tones are better protected against damage from ultraviolet rays than fairer skin types. The melanin in our skin means better protection. That built-in sunscreen means our skin will glow with youthfulness for years to come. This is why Salma Hayek, Eva Longoria, and Jennifer Lopez can rock the ageless goddess look!

Dryness is not a problem. Our skin is slightly more oily, but this is not a problem! Oil (more specifically sebum) is a natural moisturizer that keeps the skin soft and supple.

Discover Your Skin Color

Sometimes it can be tricky to determine where your skin tone falls on the Fitzpatrick scale. The simple questions below will help you figure things out. All you need to do is answer honestly and keep track of your answers.

- **What is your original hair color?**

A – Light blonde or red.

B – Medium blonde or dark blonde.

C – Light brown.

D – Medium brown.

E – Dark brown

F – Black.

- **The color of your eyes are?**

A – Light blue, light green, light gray.

B – Dark blue, dark gray, dark green.

C – Light brown or brownish-green.

D – Medium Brown.

E – Dark Brown.

F – Black (very dark brown).

- **Before you sunbathe, what color is your skin?**

A – Very light skin, pinkish, reddish.

B – Light skin, between light and beige.

C – Moderately light in winter and light tan in summer.

D – Light brown with traces of olive.

E – Brown.

F – Dark brown.

- **Any freckles?**

A – I have an abundance of freckles since very young.

B – There are quite a few freckles present.

C – I have some freckles.

D – I have afew.

E – Some that have appeared with age.

F – None at all.

- **Sunlight makes you...**

A – Turn red super quickly, without the decency of leaving a tan.

B – Burn easily, but I can tan very slightly.

C – Got a nice tan after getting burned.

D – I get a beautiful tan and I hardly get sunburn.

E – I tan easily in a short time.

F – A lick of sunlight is enough to give my skin an enviable tan.

Tally your answers. If your answers were predominantly A, your skin falls under Type I. Mostly B's are Type II. If C answers rang true for you, your skin falls under Type III. If your answers were predominantly D answers are linked to Type IV skin, Mostly E's are Type V. Lastly, predominantly F answers are linked to Type VI skin.

♥ • ♥ • ♥ • ♥ • ♥

The Skinny on SPF

Now that you know where on the Fitzpatrick Scale your skin type falls, you need to protect it from the sun's harmful rays. The shield of choice? Good old sunscreen! With so many products available, choosing the right one can be a tricky task. Fortunately, a little knowledge goes a long way. So let's demystify sun protection products once and for all.

Product labels contain a wealth of information. Sun protection products should have a number on the label. This number is known as the SPF number and indicates the level of protection the product offers. The label should also indicate if the product is broadspectrum or not. The SPF number ranges from 15 (which is low) to well over 50 (which offers maximum protection).

SPF is a scientific measure, indicating how much the risk of skin damage is lowered due to the use of sunscreen (McGill, 2018). The focus is primarily on the time UVB rays take to penetrate through the sunscreen to turn the skin red. This number is divided by the time it takes the skin to turn red without sunscreen, resulting in an SPF number. These calculations are based on a very specific amount of product that is applied to the skin. Two milligrams of product for every square centimeter of the skin surface are applied to determine the SPF number. If it takes 15 times longer to burn the skin with sunscreen than without, you've got SPF 15.

Many erroneously assume that the higher the SPF the longer one can spend in the sun. This is not quite true. Many other variables can influence the level of protection that sunscreen provides. Weather conditions, skin type, application method, and even the time of day can play a role! Most people use far too little sunscreen to start with. You will need to reapply the product every two hours, as the blocking effect wears off. If you are swimming you will need to reapply sunscreen more frequently. SPF also indicates the percentage of UV rays that are blocked. SPF 15 blocks 93% of all UVB rays, while SPF 50 blocks out 98%. Not all UV rays make the skin turn red. UVA can lead to photoaging and skin damage linked to premature aging. UVA and UVB rays are the culprits behind skin cancer, so we need to protect our skin against both. This is where we need to inspect labels carefully, because not all sunscreens protect us from UVA damage. This is why it is vital to look for a sunscreen that indicates it offers broad-spectrum or full-spectrum protection.

Tips for Using Sunscreen Effectively

Now that we have a better understanding of sunscreen, I'll share a few tips on how to get maximum protection from your product.

- I mentioned most people use too little sunscreen. Generally, one ounce is enough for a single application on the average body size. Don't forget to reapply after two hours!

- Don't rely on sunscreen alone. Hats, sunglasses, and long sleeve clothing can help to limit your exposure to UV light. These items don't have to be drab! There are many sexy, fashionable options that will provide adequate protection from the sun.

- The sun is at its most potent between 10:00 and 16:00. Try to avoid exposing yourself during these hours. Sun exposure during the midday hours is roughly four times as intense during these hours (FDA, 2018).

- Apply your sunscreen 15 minutes before venturing into the sun. If you are going for a swim, reapply the product every 40 minutes.

- Use a waterproof sunscreen when you are planning on enjoying water-bound activities.

- Lotions, creams, sprays, mousses, and gels have different application volumes. Check the label to ensure you are applying the appropriate amount.

- You'll still need sunscreen even if you avoid direct sunlight. UV rays are reflected when they hit snow, water, metal, and some other surfaces. In other words, even if you are hiding under a beach umbrella or parasol, you are still exposed to UV rays and will need sunscreen.

- Choose the right SPF for your skin. Fairer skin needs a higher SPF.

- Planning on going for a run or working up a sweat? Don't forget to reapply your sunscreen more frequently then. Sweat and the rub of clothing can remove that protective barrier quicker from your skin, leaving you unprotected.

Understanding the UV Index

One tool can help us mitigate the risk of excessive sun exposure a bit more. That tool is the UV Index (UVI). The index was developed as part of an international effort by the WHO, the United Nations Environment Programme, and the World Meteorological Organization (World Health Organization, n.d.). This educational tool was designed to reduce our risk of developing skin cancer but requires us to be proactive.

Many people plan their activities according to the weather forecast, taking special note of the temperature. Comparable to a temperature forecast, the UVI gives an estimate of the level of UV radiation one could expect. Numbers are assigned for the different levels of UV radiation. Here's a breakdown of what those numbers mean:

- **Zero to two:** It is safe to be outside.

- **Three to seven:** Use sunscreen and avoid the midday sun. If you have to go outside, seek shade whenever possible.

- **Eight:** Don't go outside. UV exposure is at its highest. Sunscreen and a hat are not negotiable. Protect yourself as much as possible and seek shade wherever you can.

UV levels can vary considerably from place to place. The time of day is also important to take note of. If you love traveling, do yourself a favor and take a peek at the UV Index before exploring your new surroundings. We often underestimate the damage the sun can do to our skin when on vacation.

· ❤ · ❤ · ❤ · ❤ · ❤ ·

Dark Skin and Cancer

Let's set the record straight: everyone can potentially develop melanoma cancer. Yes, there is a relationship between melanin and skin cancer. The relationship is one of concentration. The fairer your skin, the bigger your risk. Research indicates that the odds of Hispanics contracting the condition are one in 167, or 0.6% (American Cancer Society, 2022). In general, the risk of melanoma increases with age, but occurs more frequently in women under the age of 50 since these women are more likely to use tanning beds and lie out in the sun more frequently. The sad reality is that women under 30 remain one of the most affected age groups, and the risk only continues to increase with age. All those hours in the sun are not doing your health any favors.

There is a belief in Hispanic culture that we don't have to worry about skin cancer. We've heard it from our parents and grandparents, and while the risk is statistically lower than in Caucasians, it remains a very real and present danger. Latino families face significant barriers, with access to healthcare and adequate insurance being the biggest hurdles. This is significant! Hispanics often find out they have cancer at a very late stage, which contributes to a much higher death rate.

Only 77% of Hispanics survive five years after their diagnosis (American Cancer Society, n.d.).

The risk of contracting melanoma is much lower for Hispanics than Caucasians, but there is still a significant risk. It is estimated that up to half of Americans who live until 65 will have skin cancer at least once in their life (Borve, 2017).

Risk Factors

Early detection is a key ingredient to beating melanoma, but other risk factors come into play as well. A risk factor increases the likelihood of disease developing, and while we can control some risk factors (such as excessive exposure to sunlight), other factors (like family history) can't be changed. Having several risk factors does not mean melanoma is guaranteed to develop! Not at all. Many people with risk factors never develop the disease (American Cancer Society, 2019). Knowing the risk factors will help you take the steps needed to lower your risk of developing the disease.

- **Exposure to UV Light.** Skin cancers are mostly caused by UV rays. Apart from sunlight, there are man-made sources of UV radiation that we should be wary of. Tanning beds and sun lamps are two artificial sources of UV radiation. UV radiation is troublesome because it damages the DNA inside our skin cells. We are at risk of developing skin cancer when the areas that control cell growth and division are damaged.

- **Moles.** Most moles are harmless, but you'll need to keep an eye on them if you have many. People who have a lot of moles are associated with an increased risk of developing melanoma. Be on the lookout for atypical moles. These moles are larger than others and are unusual in shape or color. Moles can appear anywhere on the body and are often hereditary. While the chances of any particular mole turning into cancer are low, people with many atypical moles have an increased risk and will need to regularly examine their skin.

- **Being Caucasian.** Caucasians have a significantly higher risk of developing skin cancer than other people. Caucasians with natural blonde or red hair who burn or develop freckles easily are at an even higher risk.

- **Family History.** Family history plays a role in roughly a tenth of melanoma cases. When our parents, siblings, or children (first-degree relatives) develop the condition, our risk significantly increases. This is why most experts would advise individuals with a family history of melanoma to have regular skin exams. Monthly self-examinations, avid sun protection, and avoiding sources of UV radiation (like tanning beds) are simple and effective ways of reducing the risk.

- **Personal History.** Someone who has had melanoma or other types of skin cancer is at a higher risk of developing the disease.

- **Weak Immune System.** Your immune system does more than help you heal from the common cold. Our immune system is truly wonderful and can fight off cancers in the skin and organs. People who are immunocompromised or have weakened immune systems sadly fall into a higher risk category and will be more likely to develop skin cancer.

- **Aging and Gender.** The risk of developing melanoma is naturally higher for older individuals, but can affect younger people too. In fact, women under the age of 50 are actually more likely to develop the disease, presumably because younger women will spend more time bronzing their skin on the beach or on tanning beds. After 50 the tables turn and men become the high-risk group, since men routinely spend more time outside and are less likely to protect their skin with sunscreen.

- **Xeroderma Pigmentosum.** This condition is inherited and directly affects how skin cells repair damaged DNA. People with this condition are at high risk of developing skin cancer on exposed skin, especially in their youth.

Early Detection

The earlier a cancer is detected, the more treatment options are available. Any changes in the look and feel of a patch of skin, mole, blemish, or mark can divulge important clues whether cancer is developing. A new mole (or one that has changed in shape, color, and size) is one of the most important signs to look out for. When evaluating a mole, follow the ABCDE rule.

- **A – Asymmetry.** If one half of the mole or birthmark does not match the other, it's a good idea to have the mole examined by a specialist.

- **B – Border.** Jagged, uneven, or poorly defined borders are a sign that you should have a mole or birthmark checked by a specialist.

- **C – Color.** Color that is not uniform is another vital sign to be on the lookout for. Different shades of brown or black can be present. Sometimes flecks of red, white, pink, or blue can be spotted as well.

- **D – Diameter.** A pencil eraser is a handy size guide here. If the mole has a diameter that exceeds that of the average pencil eraser (roughly a quarter-inch or six millimeters), it should be checked by a specialist, although melanomas can be smaller too!

- **E – Evolution.** Moles changing in size, shape, and color are cause for concern.

Other important early warning signs include a sore that does not heal and pigment that spreads from the edge of a spot. The surrounding skin could be swollen and redness can spread beyond the edge of the mole. Changes in the surface of the mole, such as peeling, bleeding, or oozing is cause for concern.

A Word on Normal Moles

Normal moles are usually uniform in color and can be brown, tan, or black. Moles are normally round or oval in shape and can be flat against the skin or prominent. Moles usually remain constant in size, shape, and color when they develop.

Prevention

The steps to preventing melanoma are incredibly simple and can form part of your daily routine! These three steps will not eliminate all the risks, but they will significantly reduce them.

- **Limit Exposure to UV Light.** Sticking to the shade whenever possible, using sunscreen, and covering up with a hat and sunglasses are useful strategies to adopt when you are out and about. Avoiding tanning beds and artificial sources of UV light is another practical lifestyle change. Remember, UV light is harmful, irrespective if it comes from the sun or manmade sources! We should educate children on the importance of sun protection. Teaching them good skin-protecting habits from a young age will save them many troubles in the future.

- **Don't Ignore Abnormal Moles.** A routine, monthly self-examination will help you detect any abnormalities early. Follow the ABCDE rule to evaluate moles. If you spot anything out of the ordinary, err on the side of caution and have a doctor check it.

- **Bolster Your Immune System.** A weak immune system increases our risk of getting sick from all kinds of things. Eating enough fruits, veggies and healthy foods is one of the simplest ways to toughen up the immune system and protect your body.

Skin is fascinating. Identifying your skin type can reveal more than what sun protection you should use! Your skin type determines your facial care routine. In the next chapter, we'll discover more wonderful secrets your skin hides, so keep reading.

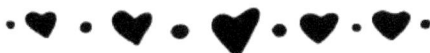

· ♥ · ♥ · ♥ · ♥ · ♥ ·

Two

Your Skin Type

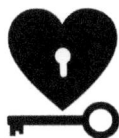

W hich organ is the largest and most complicated in the human body? The answer is quite literally wrapped all around you. It is the skin. This organ contains many specialized structures and cells, but the importance of our skin goes even deeper. The health of our skin can dictate the health of our bodies! The skin is a barrier that protects our bodies from the environment, but it does so much more! The skin plays a role in regulating our body temperature. More than that, this organ gathers sensory data from our environment. Without the skin, we would not be able to appreciate the texture of silk or sense an approaching cold spell. The skin also plays a role in the immune system. All the more reason to be kind to the skin you are in.

When we think of skin it is usually with a one-dimensional approach. We think of the layer that we can see and touch, i.e., the surface or epidermis. What many fail to realize is that a healthy glow, acne, dryness, and sweat are processed and affected by activities deep in the skin. In this regard, our skin is very similar to assembling a layered cake. Any baker will tell you that the secret to a beautiful-looking cake lies in assembling the supporting layers with care. The buttercream, icing, or fondant are merely finishing touches that enhance the cake's existing aesthetics. Neglecting the inner layers of our skin is akin to hastily assembling a layered cake: You simply won't get the result you want. This is why understanding the structure of the skin is so important!

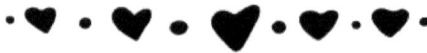

$$\cdot\,\heartsuit\cdot\heartsuit\cdot\heartsuit\cdot\heartsuit\cdot\heartsuit\cdot$$

Skin Structure

The skin has three layers. These layers are the epidermis, dermis, and subcutaneous tissue. Let's take a look at these layers in detail.

Epidermis

This is the layer that we see when applying makeup, lotions or when using cleansers. It is the outermost part of the skin and is made from epithelial tissue. These are large sheets of cells that cover the body. This layer does not have any blood vessels, and that's a good thing considering all the chemicals we are exposed to daily. This top layer is not very strong, but through secretions of various glands, it remains protected. Just under the epidermis, a membrane can be found. It is through this membrane that all the good ingredients in our creams and serums must travel to reach the deeper layers of our skin. The epidermis is thickest in the soles of our feet and the palms.

When we dive a bit deeper into the wonderful structure that is the epidermis, we discover several layers hidden within.

- **Basal Layer.** This layer is characterized by germ cells that are constantly dividing. These cells (stem cells or germ cells) produce cytokines and interferons. These proteins are vital to the healthy functioning of the immune system. These proteins play a crucial role in the body's immune response.

- **Spinous Layer.** Special cells known as polygonal keratinocytes are found in this layer. As these cells migrate towards the surface of our skin, something special happens. These cells undergo structural and biochemical changes. Under the microscope, these cells seem to have "spines" which is where the name is derived from. The spines serve as a bridge between cells, allowing for adhesion and communication between cells.

- **Granular Layer.** These cells have a peculiar shape to them. They are wide in the middle and taper towards the ends. In biology, this shape is referred to as a spindle shape. This layer plays an important role in the barrier function of our skin.

- **Stratum Lucidum.** A special layer that is only found in our palms and the soles of our feet.

- **Stratum Corneum.** The outermost layer of the epidermis that is in direct contact with the environment is mainly composed of keratin and filaggrin. These flat polyhedral cells are constantly shed from the surface of the skin.

In addition to all these layers, the epidermis contains three very special cells. Melanocytes produce melanin and are responsible for the color of our skin. Langerhans cells are our skin's first line of defense, while Merkel cells are not fully understood. It is believed that Merkel cells play a role in the sensation of touch.

Dermis

This thick layer of connective tissue is located just under the epidermis and contains lymphatic vessels and blood vessels, nerve endings, sebaceous glands, and hair follicles. There are many specialized cells and structures that call the dermis home. When we get a papercut, it is this layer that gets hurt. Within the dermis, there are two layers.

- **Papillary Dermis.** The touch receptors can be found here and this layer is rich in blood vessels and nerves.

- **Reticular Dermis.** This deeper layer houses a dense network of collagen, hair follicles, sweat glands, and sebaceous glands.

Subcutaneous Tissue

The deepest part of the skin, the subcutaneous cellular tissue, is mainly made from fatty connective tissue and bands of collagen. We can think of fatty connective tissues as multifunctional shock-absorbers. Apart from shielding delicate nerve, lymphatic, and blood systems, fatty tissues insulate against heat loss and can store energy and water. The thickness of this layer varies. You'll have a much thinner layer in your hands, compared to the thicker layer found in the buttocks or legs. The skin is truly assembled like a multi-layered rainbow cake, with each layer having a unique characteristic.

· ♥ · ♥ · ♥ · ♥ · ♥ ·

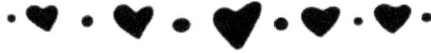

Functions of the Skin

The way the skin is structured is the same for all races. The only variable is the amount of pigment that each person's melanocytes produce. When we zoom in on how the skin is structured and functions, it can become a unifying force, highlighting everything we have in common with our fellow man.

- Everyone's skin offers two types of protection: mechanical and thermal. In other words, our skin keeps us safe from the environment and helps to regulate body temperature.

- The skin protects against infection. Bacteria have a hard time penetrating healthy skin. Even if some bacteria manage to slip past the outer barriers of the skin, they still have to contend with the Langerhans cells.

- The skin is our largest sensory organ. Just imagine how different life would be if we could not feel vibrations, pain, or temperature. There'd be a lot more accidents and deaths guaranteed.

- Interestingly, the skin functions as a bit of a blood reserve. One-tenth of our total blood volume can be found in the blood vessels of the skin when we are at rest (Rodriguez,

2017). With so much blood circulating our skin, it becomes clear why dermatologists often say that good skin starts within.

- When our bodies are undernourished, the subcutaneous tissue becomes an important energy deposit. It is an age-old survival adaptation to fuel our hungry brains (Duke University, 2019).

- Lastly, the skin synthesizes Vitamin D and produces sweat and sebum in every human being.

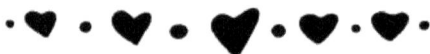

· ♥ · ♥ · ♥ · ♥ · ♥ ·

Types of Facial Skin

There are different ways of classifying skin types. The Fitzpatrick Scale (discussed in the previous chapter) is a useful tool to find out what SPF you should be using, but we can't rely on it alone to determine our overall skin care regimen. Doing so is akin to using a hammer when you need a needle. For this reason, skin is classified differently from a cosmetic perspective.

Each skin type is special and will need a different approach to care. Genetics play a role in determining your skin type, but other variables such as age and the environment exert a significant influence as well.

The standard classification of skin types into normal, oily, combination, dry, and sensitive skin types should not be entirely unfamiliar.

You may have seen these descriptions on bottles of moisturizers and cleansers, but what exactly does it mean to have "normal" or "combination" skin?

Normal Skin

This skin type is often described as having a regular texture and no imperfections (CuídatePlus Editorial Office, 2017). The skin typically has a smooth appearance and uniform tone. It is a very low-maintenance skin type, but can become dry if neglected.

Oily Skin

Individuals with this skin type would have a shiny appearance all over their faces. This shiny appearance is due to the high production of sebum. The usual challenges with this skin type are blackheads and pimples. This skin type produces more sebum and will require a specific care routine. Regular exfoliation is important to keep the skin smooth and free from dirt. Oily skin can be caused by a variety of factors like hormonal imbalance, genetics, climate, age, lifestyle, and diet. The best way to turn things around for this skin type is to get to the root of the problem and follow an appropriate skincare plan.

Combination Skin

This skin type is a bit of a hybrid, combining normal and oily skin. The T-zone which consists of the forehead, nose, and chin tends to be oily, while the cheeks remain dry. Combination skin is tricky to care for due to the mix of characteristics, but there is no need to be despondent. A weekly exfoliation and nourishing mask can work wonders!

A number of factors contribute to combination skin, but most of the time it comes down to genetics. Seasonal changes and the skin care products you are using can exacerbate the problem. Products containing harsh ingredients tend to dry the cheeks and trigger more oil production in the T-zone. To help bring balance to the skin, try to avoid products that include these ingredients:

- Alcohol, menthol, witch hazel, or denatured alcohol, which is a common ingredient in toners.

- Overly abrasive scrubs.

- Strong scents. Skincare products that have a strong, lasting scent can irritate the skin, regardless if the fragrance is natural or synthetic in origin.

Dry Skin

People who have this skin type often experience a feeling of tightness. A lack of moisture in the skin gives rise to tightness and an older appearance. Dry skin types are quite sensitive to climate changes and can have a dull appearance and rough feel. Good hydration is key to treating dry skin.

Dehydrated Skin

Often confused for dry skin, dehydrated skin is a sign that you need to drink more water and make some lifestyle changes. A simple test to find out if your skin is dehydrated is to lightly pinch a portion of your skin around the cheek area. If you notice wrinkling and if the skin doesn't bounce back immediately after you let go, chances are you are dehydrated. A dermatologist or aesthetician can help you classify your skin if you are unsure. Remember, dry skin essentially points to a lack of oils, whereas dehydrated skin indicates a lack of water.

Sensitive Skin

Sensitive skin is very reactive. This skin type will react to environmental stimuli that would not bother normal skin. The reaction is usually accompanied by discomfort, tightness, redness, or itching. When the protective function of our skin is compromised, sensitive skin is the result and will need a greater degree of care. In this category, we will find photosensitive and hypersensitive skin.

- **Photosensitive Skin.** Photosensitivity, which is often referred to as a "sun allergy" is an immune system response triggered by sunlight (Benedetti, 2022). People with this condition typically develop itchy eruptions, redness, and inflammation on exposed skin. Diagnosis is based on a medical evaluation.

- **Hypersensitive Skin.** Also known as very sensitive skin, this common and unpleasant condition is characterized by dry skin, irritation, eczema, pimples, redness, or sensations of burning and stinging (Eucerin, n.d.-b). Hypersensitive skin is the result of a compromised skin barrier and will need special care. Certain fabrics and dyes can irritate this skin type, but generally, the triggers differ from person to person.

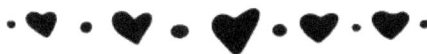

· ♥ · ♥ · ♥ · ♥ · ♥ ·

Determining Your Skin Type

Selecting the right skincare routine boils down to knowing your skin type. When we use products that are not designed for our skin type, the efficacy of those products are reduced. Fortunately, this easy quiz will help you set things straight. Write down the letter corresponding to your answer and check it against the results at the end of the quiz.

- **When you wake up, your face looks...**

A – Shiny and oily all over.

B – A little shiny.

C – Oily on the nose, forehead, and chin.

D – A little dull.

- **After cleansing your skin it feels...**

A – Like I need to wash my face again.

B – Great!

C – Tight in the forehead, nose, and chin areas.

D – Dry and tight all over my face.

- **How does your skin feel three hours after cleansing?**

A – It feels like I haven't washed my face at all.

B – My skin still feels good.

C – My nose, chin, and forehead could do with some cleansing again.

D – My whole face feels dry.

- **Take a close look at the surface of the skin. What do you see?**

A – I see a lot of bumps.

B – There is tender and thickened skin.

C – I see bumps, but there is tender skin too.

D – The skin is thin and dry.

- **What is your experience with your skin?**

A – My skin always seems to be shiny and acne-prone.

B – My skin is mostly hydrated and free from problems.

C – My skin ranges from oily to normal.

D – My skin tends to be dry and sensitive, prone to irritations.

- **Take a look at your pores. What do they look like?**

A – I see visible, large, and closed pores.

B – I hardly notice them!

C – The pores on my chin, nose, and forehead are visible.

D – I can't see my pores.

- **During the day your face is...**

A – Gray or yellowish in color.

B – Pinkish.

C – My forehead, nose, and chin always have a different color from the rest of my face.

D – Pale and without a glow.

- **During the summer, how much does your skin darken?**

A – I can gradually tan without burning.

B – I tan easily but end up slightly red.

C – I can gradually tan, but end up with a sunburn.

D – My skin burns very easily and turns immediately red.

- **When you do your makeup, how long does it last?**

A – I need touch-ups every three or four hours.

B – I only need a touch-up around noon, then it lasts all day.

C – My makeup lasts half a day.

D – My makeup lasts all day without needing any touch-ups.

- **During puberty you had...**

A – Acne that still pesters me!

B – Acne that disappeared after puberty.

C – Some pimples, but it was manageable.

D – No acne at all.

Take a look at your answers. Count all the A's, B's, C's, and D's. If your answers were mostly A, you have oily skin. Mostly B reveals that you have normal skin. If the answers in C spoke to you, you have combination skin. Mostly D answers will reveal that you have dry skin.

· ♥ · ♥ · ♥ · ♥ · ♥ ·

Changes in Your Skin Type

Your skin type is not set in stone. Yes, it is true that your skin type is genetically determined, but it does not mean it will remain unchanged. One such example is oily skin turning into dry skin as we age. This is a change that is normally triggered by menopause when our sebaceous glands become less active. The skin can react to hormones and environmental changes, so it is important to adjust your skincare routine when needed. Let's take a peek at some changes our skin can undergo.

Skin Becomes Drier

Dry skin often feels itchy and can develop a scaly and red appearance. Cold temperatures in autumn and winter tend to dry the skin out more. It is best to use hydrating cleansers during this time. A moisturizer rich in ceramides can help to seal in moisture to keep dryness away. If dryness persists you may need to use a humidifier to introduce some moisture into your environment if possible.

Skin Becomes Oilier

Oily skin often has a shiny appearance and a heavy feel. If you notice your skin is turning oilier, relax. The change is temporary and likely due to hormonal changes. The skin can become oilier during the menstrual cycle as hormone levels change. Changes in hormone levels temporarily stimulate the sebaceous glands to produce more sebum than normal. To combat excess oiliness cleanse twice daily. Choose products that have absorbent ingredients like bentonite clay to keep the face matte and remove impurities gently. Follow up with a light, non-greasy serum and moisturizer to lock the goodness in your skin. Gel formulations work the best.

Skin Becomes Dry and Oily

Perhaps you have noticed your T-zone becoming shiny, or your cheeks getting drier. The change in seasons usually triggers this change in our skin and is temporary. When certain parts of our skin become oilier it is best to treat the skin like combination skin until it returns to normal. Opt for a sulfate-free cleanser. It reduces oiliness but is gentle enough not to strip the skin of all moisture. Follow up with light serums and moisturizers that contain hyaluronic acid to lock in moisture without introducing greasiness. Hyaluronic acid is quite an interesting ingredient. It absorbs up to a thousand times its own weight in water! These moisture-retaining properties are what make hyaluronic acid so effective to fill in wrinkles and fine lines.

External and internal factors, such as the environment and hormones, can influence the skin. When you notice a change in your skin, stop and ask yourself:

- Was it a change in the seasons that triggered the change?

- Are you more stressed than usual?

- Did you use a different product (like a lower SPF sunscreen)?

- Has your diet been lacking any essential nutrients?

If the change is due to internal factors (diet, stress, hormones) we have to make changes in our daily routine. Try to relax more if you are stressed and make any dietary changes that are needed to ensure you eat a healthy, balanced diet. Having an appropriate skincare routine for your skin type is crucial to maintaining a youthful, radiant appearance. In the next chapter, I'll share more skincare secrets with you!

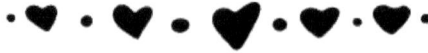

· ♥ · ♥ · ♥ · ♥ · ♥ ·

Three
The Why of Facial Skincare

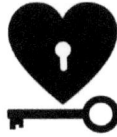

F acial hygiene is an important step in maintaining a radiant appearance. It is a mistake to think a quick splash to remove the *legañas* is enough. If we are not kind to our skin the results will show years from now! The skin releases more oil during the night (Saludalia, n.d.). That is why a good, daily cleansing routine is vital. Moisturizing night creams tend to be thicker than those used during the day, so they need to be washed off in the morning to prevent future skin problems from cropping up.

Doing a complete facial cleanse before your shower is a great way to show your skin that extra bit of love, especially if you have oily skin. For best results use a mild cleansing cream, especially on the T-zone. Cleansing creams should be free from detergents, as these can strip the skin and cause irritation. There are many options ranging from moisturizing milks, gels, and gentle soaps.

After the skin has been cleansed, apply a toner that is suitable for your skin type. The toner helps to clean any remaining dirt from the face and closes the pores. Keep in mind that facial hygiene is an important step in controlling oil production, removing dead skin cells, eliminating blackheads, and preventing wrinkles. Regular, daily cleansing is especially important if you love to wear makeup or live in an urban area. A regular cleanse will help remove pollutants, grease, makeup residue, and dust from your face to keep the pores free from clogs for a radiant appearance.

You may be surprised to learn that the reasons we should take care of our skin are closely intertwined with skin function. In the previous chapter we learned about these functions, now let's take a look at how they link up with skincare.

- *Skincare keeps your armor healthy.* The skin is our first line of defense, our armor that protects our bodies from damage and disease. Keeping the armor in tip-top shape not only allows it to protect our bodies better, but keeps us looking beautiful and healthy.

- *Staves off premature aging.* Aging is inevitable, but showing our age early on does not have to be. Skincare helps us to delay the visible effects that the ravages of time can have, helping us retain a youthful appearance for longer.

- *Keeps the skin hydrated.* Exposure to the sun without proper protection can result in dryness. When we have a good skincare routine in place, with the appropriate sunscreen and moisturizer, dryness can be avoided altogether.

- *Preventing skin cancer.* This is a huge reason to religiously care for your skin! By avoiding sunburn and nourishing the skin we can drastically reduce our risk of contracting skin cancer.

- *Beautiful skin is a reflection of good health.* Good physical health and a healthy immune system are attributes we often assign to people who have healthy, luminous skin. Healthy skin also gives us a confidence boost, so there is truth in that old saying: "When we look good, we feel good."

- *Reducing the appearance of spots.* Prevention is key, as many spots are caused by exposure to the sun without protection.

Skincare runs a little deeper than simply looking and feeling drop-dead gorgeous. It empowers us to face the world a little more confidently and gives our largest organ a much-needed helping hand. With all the care products available on the market it can be overwhelming, but I will show you how they work and explain the characteristics they should meet to be suitable for your skin type.

· ❤ · ❤ · ❤ · ❤ · ❤ ·

Facial Cleansers

Everyone is guilty of forgetting to cleanse their face from time to time. When we use powerful, active ingredients without cleansing the skin first, we are essentially flushing money down the drain. Cleansing removes dirt, makeup, and other impurities from the skin improving the functioning of your other skincare products. Knowing when to double cleanse and what mistakes to avoid can go a long way to improving the skin's immediate appearance.

Double Cleanse

One of the most valuable lessons we can take from K-beauty is the nightly double cleanse! Korean women take extra care to remove all impurities before applying treatment products and the results are stunning. The good news is this Korean beauty secret is suitable for all skin types. It's not about aggressive cleansing, but more about doing it in two steps following your skin's needs (Nast, 2021b).

Removing Makeup Effectively

Makeup is a useful tool to highlight our natural beauty, but it can be notoriously difficult to remove. Many of us rely on wipes, but this is not an effective step. To remove makeup properly, you'll need to find a makeup remover that is suited for your skin type. Choose an oil-based formulation, as oil dissolves dirt extremely well and does not strip the skin of moisture. Oil-based formulations are suitable for all skin types. Micellar water, on the other hand, is not suitable as a base cleanser. Use micellar water in your second cleansing step when double cleansing in the evening, or for the morning cleanse.

Choosing the Right Product for Your Skin Type

Foams, milks, gels... it's all a matter of taste, right? The answer is not as cut and dried as one might expect. While we tend to use more of a product that we like, there is a method behind all the madness in the cosmetic aisle. I'll let you in on a little secret:

- Micellar water is used to cleanse sensitive skin.

- Foams and gels are best suited for combination skin.

- Cleansing milks and dry skin are best friends.

Keep in mind that ingredients do matter though. If you have dry skin but prefer to use foam, opt for moisturizing ingredients. Oily skin types can use micellar water with great success if it contains oil-regulating ingredients.

Solid soaps are an option as well, especially if you are looking to adopt a zero-waste routine. The most important thing is to look for a suitable formulation for your skin type. If you can find a soap with a pH of 5, even better! The pH of the skin is normally 4.7. A thin barrier on the surface of the skin, known as the acid mantle, helps to maintain this pH balance. The main purpose of the acid mantle is to protect the skin from environmental factors, but when we disturb this barrier by using harsh products, irritation and premature aging can ensue (Mukherjee, 2019).

Ingredients That Matter

Let's take a deep dive into the ingredients label on your cleanser. Chances are there are some interesting-sounding names on the label, but are they suitable for your skin type? This quick reference guide will help you select the cleansers with the most beneficial ingredients for your skin type.

- ***Combination and Oily Skin:*** Look for ingredients that regulate sebum production. Ingredients that love these skin types include salicylic acid, tea tree oil, niacinamide, green tea, and alpha-hydroxy acids.

- **Sensitive Skin:** These skin types need soothing, decongestant, and anti-redness ingredients. Sensitive skin loves allantoin, aloe vera, centella asiatica, niacinamide, turmeric, and green tea.

- **Dry Skin:** Here we need ingredients that will reinforce the protective barrier of the skin. Moisturizing ingredients like glycols, panthenol, urea, allantoin, hydroxy acids (more specifically lactic acid), and hyaluronic acid are excellent to use for dry skin.

- **Normal Skin:** This skin type is very easy-going. Any regular cleanser aimed at normal skin will be suitable to maintain the balance of your skin.

Cleansing Sins

Acquiring a cleanser with skin-loving ingredients is the first step to a more youthful, radiant you. Next, you need to keep that momentum going by avoiding some of the most common mistakes we all make on our journey to fabulous skin.

- **Relying Excessively on Wipes.** This cleansing sin happens more frequently than we care to admit. Wipes are convenient after all! Sadly, wipes can't be considered a true cleanser. They are great to use in specific situations, but should not form the foundation of our skincare routine.

- *Using the Wrong Products.* Simply relying on a cleanser to remove sunscreen and makeup is not effective. A cleanser is not formulated to remove makeup effectively. In this situation, it is best to double cleanse. Start with the makeup remover first and follow up with a skin-loving cleanser.

- *Relying on Astringent Products.* Oily and combination skin are not friends with astringent products. These products strip the skin of lipids, leaving it feeling dry and tight. For best results refer to the ingredients guide. Your skin will thank you!

- *Rinsing with Hot or Cold Water.* Temperature extremes are not friendly to the skin and can cause discomfort. Show your skin love and opt to use pleasantly warm water instead.

- *Roughhousing Your Face with a Towel.* Instinctively grabbing the towel and wiping the face can encourage the formation of wrinkles and reintroduces dirt onto the skin. The correct way to dry your face is to pat the skin dry with a towel that is reserved for use on your face.

- *Skipping the Toner.* Toners are often an optional step, so it's not exactly a sin to skip them, but sensitive, oily, and combination skin types may find benefit from adding a toner to their routine. Toners stimulate and refresh the skin, promoting good hygiene. Furthermore, toners contribute to improved circulation and can help to maintain the muscle tone of the skin. The result? Firmer and more beautiful skin.

- ***Assuming Facial Cleansing Brushes Removes Makeup.*** Electronic facial cleansing brushes are wonderful to stimulate circulation in the skin, but these brushes were not designed to remove makeup and should be used in the second step of cleansing only. Be cautious when using these brushes on sensitive skin types as they may irritate.

Cleanser Tips

How well you cleanse your face influences the efficacy of your other skincare products. I'll share four tips to help you get the most out of your cleanser. Go ahead and try them, you'll see and feel the difference after a single wash.

- Store everything you need in one place. Running around with a wet face in search of a towel is hardly an effective way to start your skincare routine. Keep everything you need (towels and products) close at hand. It is a great time saver!

- Massage while you cleanse. When we massage the face in small, ascending circles we stimulate circulation. This is a useful strategy to reduce puffiness under the eyes. Better circulation leads to better nourishment for the skin. Regular massages while you cleanse, can improve circulation for healthier-looking skin.

- Exfoliate your skin. This removes product buildup along with dead skin cells. Never use an exfoliator on dry skin. It is recommended to rub the product in ascending circles for a massage benefit.

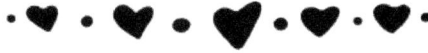

•❤•❤•❤•❤•❤•

Eye Contour

The eye contour is a very fragile area and should be handled with care. The skin is extremely thin in this area and requires gentle products and a gentle touch. Eye contour cream helps to improve circulation in the area and reduces the appearance of wrinkles. A common mistake we tend to make is to assume that regular moisturizer is good enough for the eye area, but eye contour creams are specifically formulated to be easily absorbed by the delicate, thin skin around the eye. Regular moisturizer simply won't cut it. In fact, using products that are not designed for the eye area can encourage fine lines and wrinkles to appear much sooner!

Did you know it is recommended to begin using eye contour at the age of 20? That is because our skin's needs change as we age. When we are in our early 20s, contour creams enriched with Vitamin E are best. After 25, select an eye contour cream that contains hyaluronic acid or Vitamin C to stave off the signs of premature aging. More mature skin will benefit most from eye contour that is rich in antioxidants. The idea is to stimulate collagen production. Are your eyes tired and puffy? Eye contour creams formulated to deeply moisturize can help. These creams can reduce puffiness and dark circles. Select a non-greasy formulation.

Not all ingredients are good for your eye area! Scrutinize the label and avoid any products that contain alcohol, retinoic acid, salicylic acid, or urea. These ingredients can be quite aggressive and are not suitable to use on the delicate eye area.

Application Technique

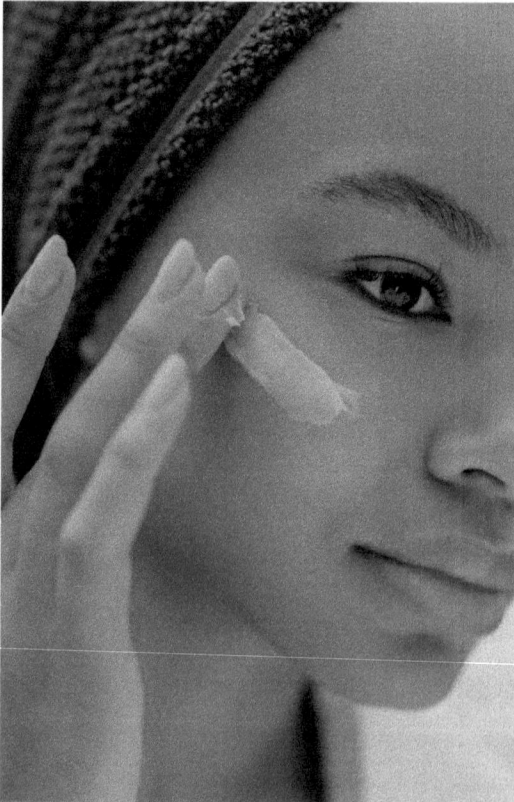

Application technique is as important as the quality of your eye contour. Incorrect application technique not only wastes the product, but can encourage fine lines to develop. Fortunately, the eye contour is not complicated to apply!

- After completing the cleansing step, place a small amount of eye contour on the back of your hand. The size of a rice grain is the correct amount of product to use.

- Using your ring finger, gently apply the product to the eye area in a circular motion. Soft and gentle is the key! You want the product to melt into your skin.

- Repeat the application every morning and night for fabulously nourished skin.

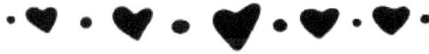

· ♥ · ♥ · ♥ · ♥ · ♥ ·

Facial Scrub

Exfoliate weekly to keep skin care products working optimally. Exfoliating removes dead skin cells, encourages cell renewal, and can restore the skin's softness. Unlocking gorgeous skin is just a facial scrub away. Product selection and use really make a difference here.

If you have combination skin, search the label for skin-purifying ingredients. Salicylic acid, eucalyptus, zinc, and clay are good options. Charcoal and salicylic acid are useful to get rid of blackheads deep in the skin. If you have a pronounced blackhead and acne problem, opt for a leave-on exfoliant containing beta hydroxy acid.

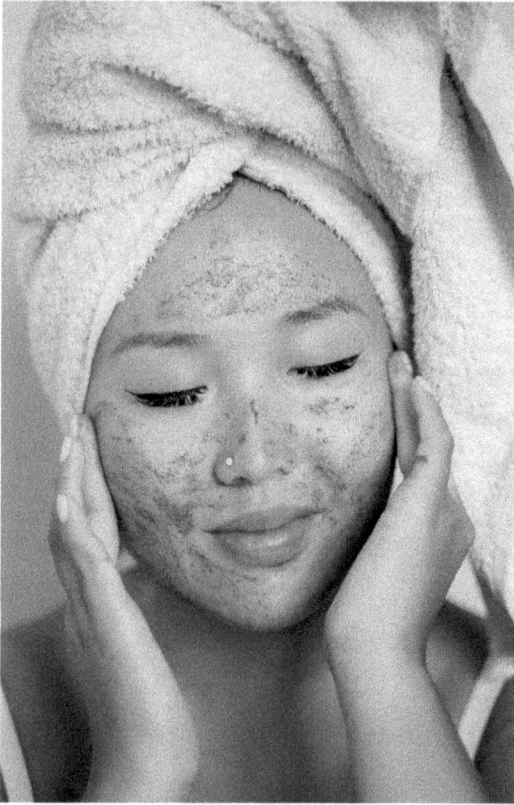

Apart from scrutinizing the label, you need to test the scrub on the back of your hand to ensure it is gentle enough for your face. Even if the ingredients are wonderful, they may be too harsh for facial use. If a scrub feels remotely scratchy it is not suitable for facial use.

The best scrubs to use for the face will contain finely milled, round particles. These ingredients exfoliate effectively without scratching the face. Scrubs containing ground-up shells, volcanic rock, and fruit pits are unsuitable for use on your face. When we use harsh scrubs regularly, we risk creating flaky patches, redness, and sensitivity in the skin. This issue can be exacerbated if the scrub contains a fragrance.

Many scrubs leave a tingling sensation on the skin. Many women are led to believe that this tingling is a sign of the product working. Sadly, this belief is a bit far from the truth. Tingling is a sign of irritation. Many scrubs include ingredients like menthol and peppermint in their formulations. These ingredients leave a cooling sensation on the skin, but can be unsuitable for use on the face. As a rule of thumb, try to avoid scrubs containing these ingredients.

A common misconception is that natural ingredients like salt and fruit pits are best to use. While these ingredients make a wonderful body scrub, it is hardly suitable for use on your delicate facial skin. If you have your heart set on natural ingredients look for scrubs containing jojoba beads, oatmeal, rice bran, or silica. These ingredients are far more gentle and effective, especially when the formula contains soothing and hydrating ingredients. It is best to steer clear of sugar scrubs, they are not a healthy option. Sensitive skin will find the most benefit from natural ingredients and dissolving beads. Dissolving beads gently remove dead skin cells without any abrasiveness to minimize the risk of irritation.

The Difference Between Scrubs and Leave-on Exfoliants

Scrubs and leave-on exfoliants are not the same. Think of scrubs as jewelry polish. They make the surface beautiful, but can't remove deep-seated tarnish or rust from your favorite jewelry items. In much the same vein, scrubs can't remove built-up layers of sun damage or correct the pore lining. This is where leave-on exfoliants containing alpha hydroxy acid or beta hydroxy acid shine. These products can penetrate deep into the skin to address white bumps, blemishes, and thick built-up layers of dead skin. Beta hydroxy acid has another advantage. It can exfoliate inside the pore, improving pore function and reducing blackhead problems (Begoun, n.d.). Scrubs and leave-on exfoliants are complementary products, so feel free to use both.

Using Facial Scrubs the Right Way

The efficacy of your products largely depends on correct usage. Facial scrubs should only be applied to the forehead, nose, and cheeks. Spread the product evenly, from the forehead to the temples and down the face. Next, gently rub the product on the bridge of your nose towards the tip. From the wings of your nose, use small circular movements to rub the scrub as you move down your cheeks, jawline, and chin. Be gentle with your movements, there is no need to rub vigorously. Finally, rinse with lukewarm water. Follow up with your preferred moisturizer. Always remember to wet your face before applying the scrub and use a product that is formulated for your skin type.

Here's a pro beauty tip: Use your facial scrub in the shower! The water vapor will encourage your pores to open, making the scrub more effective.

When using scrubs, be careful of over-exfoliating. When we use scrubs too often we can disturb the skin's natural balance, leaving it feeling dry and tight.

·❤·❤·❤·❤·❤·

Facial Toner

Early versions of facial toners were very astringent, containing ingredients like witch hazel and alcohol (Nast, 2021c). These toners were notorious for causing irritation and aggravating skin conditions. Modern toners are far more gentle and typically contain ingredients like hyaluronic acid, aloe vera, glycerin, and chamomile to nourish and restore the skin.

Toners form a crucial step in the double cleansing routine and help to remove any impurities that your cleanser may have missed. On top of providing a deep clean, toners containing hydroxy acids and antioxidants gently firm the skin for a deliciously smooth texture. When selecting your toner, pay attention to the ingredients. Not all ingredients are suitable for your skin type!

- *Dry Skin and Mature Skin:* Look for toners containing glycerin and hyaluronic acid. These gentle ingredients retain moisture in the skin while giving you all the benefits associated with toners.

- *For Acne-prone and Oily Skin:* Toners with salicylic acid and tea tree oil are a good choice. These ingredients regulate oil production, improve hyperpigmentation, and can reduce the appearance of scars.

- *Normal and Combination Skin:* Toners with coenzyme Q10, hyaluronic acid, glycerin, and vitamin C are good choices.

Using a toner is a nice step to include in your beauty routine, but you can omit it if your routine is minimalist. If you do opt to use a toner, remember to apply it correctly. Use a clean cotton pad to gently apply the product to your skin. Allow your skin to fully absorb the product before continuing with the rest of your beauty routine. It is best to use toners in the morning and evening after cleansing the skin.

·♥·♥·♥·♥·♥·

Serum

Serums are a wonderful product to use right before you apply your moisturizer. These concentrated products are always applied in small amounts and usually with a dropper. The active ingredients in the product will not only deeply nourish your skin, but also boost the effects of the cream that follows (Nast, 2021a).

A rule of thumb when using multiple products is to apply them from thinnest to thickest. After cleansing, we would tone the skin, apply serum, moisturizing cream, and finally sunscreen. We apply thin products first to aid easy absorption into the skin.

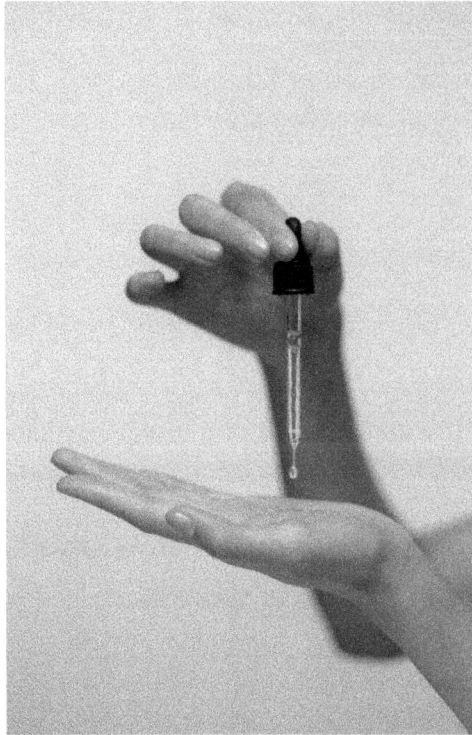

Serums are applied to the face and neck. Typically we apply a few drops to the hands and spread the product evenly over the face and neck. Alternatively, if the serum has a pipette we have the option of applying the product directly to the face. Use three to four drops at most. This may seem too little, but bear in mind that serum is highly concentrated. A little goes a very long way! It is not necessary to heat a serum. Doing so will not enhance the effectiveness and there is no evidence to support this practice.

When to Use Serums

Serums are unfairly associated only with anti-aging treatments. They are much more versatile than this one-dimensional approach will have us believe. Furthermore, there is no ideal or preferred age at which we should start using serums. A teenager can use serum rich in hyaluronic acid to reduce the side effects of acne treatments. Generally, for anti-aging benefits serums can be used from the age of 25 onwards when the production of elastin and collagen begins to slow down. This handy general age guide will help you choose the correct serum.

- In our twenties, it is best to select a product with hyaluronic acid to deeply hydrate the layers of the skin.

- In our thirties, serums with Vitamin C will help prevent and treat expression lines and wrinkles.

- From our forties onwards, Vitamin A (retinol) becomes an important ingredient to stimulate cell renewal.

- As we mature and reach our fifties, DMAE becomes the skin-firming ingredient of choice.

A Serum for Every Need

Contrary to popular belief, skin type does not influence the serum you should use. Serums are selected solely for their active ingredients and the effects they can achieve, such as skin firming or wrinkle reduction. The reference guide below will help you find the right serum for your needs.

- *Serums with Vitamin C:* These serums brighten the skin and counteract free radical damage.

- *Anti-aging:* Containing powerful antioxidants, these products stimulate collagen and elastin production to eliminate expression lines and reduce the appearance of wrinkles.

- *Repairing Serums:* These products are used at night and are formulated to boost cell activity, resulting in a rested and healthy-looking skin in the morning.

- *Reshaping Serums:* Designed to fill in wrinkles and redefine the face, these products produce visible lifting effects.

- *Firming Serums:* These are formulated with mature skin in mind. Firming serums improve skin firmness for a youthful countenance.

- *Moisturizing Serums:* Typically containing hyaluronic acid, these serums deeply moisturize the skin.

- *Anti-spot:* Created to treat pigmentation and irregular skin tone, these serums are highly effective in reducing the appearance of dark spots with consistent use.

- *Eye Contour:* Treat the eye contour with powerful ingredients to reduce expression lines, and reduce the appearance of bags and dark circles.

- *Acne:* Serums formulated to treat acne remove marks, unclog pores, and refine skin texture.

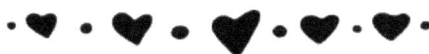

· ♥ · ♥ · ♥ · ♥ · ♥ ·

Dry Skin Cream

Creams for dry skin need to contain nutrients that hold water inside the skin. With the consistent and correct application over time, these ingredients will lead to a healthier appearing skin. There is no need to feel embarrassed if you have dry skin, anyone can get it. Dry skin can become a lifelong battle if we don't take steps to nip the condition in the bud (Zonadamas, 2021).

Treating Very Dry Skin

Abnormally dry skin is a condition that is sometimes called *Xerosis cutis*. The name comes from the Greek word "*Xero*" which means "dry." Treatments should contain ingredients that are humectant, moisturizing, and lipid-replenishing.

Humectants, like silicones, do not have a strong odor and are not comedogenic, i.e. they don't clog the pores to create blackheads. You'll find silicones in many fat-free formulations. Silicones give beauty products a smooth and silky finish that feels luxurious on the skin. Apart from improving the feel of beauty products, these little molecules fill in cracks and crevices in the skin. The result? A smoother-looking and feeling skin!

Moisturizing ingredients create a barrier layer. For this reason hyaluronic acid is used in many skincare products. This powerful ingredient has excellent moisturizing properties and restores the skin's flexibility and elasticity.

Lipid replenishers give dry skin formulations consistency and cohesion. They can improve the skin in many ways and have anti-inflammatory, antimicrobial and immunogenic properties. Search the label for linoleic acid, gamma-linolenic or arachidic. These ingredients are derived from vegetable sources like evening primrose, jojoba, shea, olive, wheat germ, and sunflower oils. Other skin-loving ingredients to be on the lookout for are aloe vera and oatmeal. These ingredients have moisturizing and anti-inflammatory properties and can prevent itchiness.

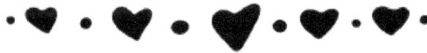

· ♥ · ♥ · ♥ · ♥ · ♥ ·

Steps to Care for Dry Skin

Take a few minutes to care for your skin to keep dry skin away. Consistency is key to keeping dry skin under control, and the order in which you apply products matters. Your daily dry skin care routine should look something like this:

- Cleansing the skin twice daily (morning and night).

- Applying toner to balance the pH.

- Applying serum. This is a vital step! The serum penetrates the skin deeply and boosts the functioning of your moisturizer.

- Following up with a moisturizer. The product should be

formulated for dry skin to prevent water loss. Look for a moisturizer that is rich in vegetable oils, Vitamin E, and hyaluronic acids.

- Lastly, applying sunscreen. Use an SPF suitable for your skin type as determined by the Fitzpatrick Scale.

Don't forget to include the other healthy skin habits we've already discussed, like drinking enough water and removing makeup with the correct products. These steps will help to retain moisture to leave you with soft, supple skin.

Evaluating Dry Skin Products

Selecting the right product for dry skin can be tricky. Some formulations trigger allergic reactions and inflammation. If you find yourself experiencing allergic reactions easily it is best to consult your dermatologist for guidance. In most cases, a hypoallergenic product will be recommended. These products are typically free from fragrance, color, and other common irritants. For a product to be truly considered hypoallergenic it needs to fulfill two conditions:

- It should not contain ingredients that triggered an allergic reaction in one percent of the population over the last five years. The guidelines are quite strict and at least 1,000 patients have to be studied before an ingredient is considered hypoallergenic.

- Search the label. If it contains any ingredients for which there is no published data over the last five years, the product can not be considered hypoallergenic.

A good product for dry skin will contain antioxidants. These ingredients protect our skin cells from the damage caused by free radicals and slow visible signs of aging. Skin-loving antioxidants include Vitamin E, Vitamin C, retinol, niacinamide, and flavonoids. These nutrients are explored in deeper detail in chapter eight. Each of these ingredients has a slightly different function which I will touch on below.

- *Vitamin E:* Dry, brittle and sensitive skin benefits from Vitamin E's ability to regenerate the skin.

- *Retinol:* Used to improve the appearance of the skin and helps to trigger cell renewal.

- *Vitamin C:* This natural antioxidant actively fights the aging process and helps to rebuild cell tissues.

- *Niacinamide:* Helps to improve blood circulation and reduces the appearance of fine lines, wrinkles, and blemishes.

- *Flavonoids:* These ingredients help to protect the body and are naturally found in a variety of fruits and vegetables.

- *Resveratrol:* Plays a role in firming the skin and enhancing collagen production. This ingredient is also anti-inflammatory.

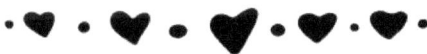

· ♥ · ♥ · ♥ · ♥ · ♥ ·

Facial Depigmenting Cream

Treatments in this category typically have their own lingua franca, making the task of selecting the correct product for your needs quite daunting. Before we dive into the deeper mechanics of these creams, we need to touch on what depigmenting creams are.

Depigmenting creams go by many names. Descriptive words like brightening, lightening, whitening, fading, or bleaching can often be spotted on the label. These products are cosmetic treatments that contain active ingredients to inhibit the production of melanin, therefore lightening the skin (Navarro, 2021a).

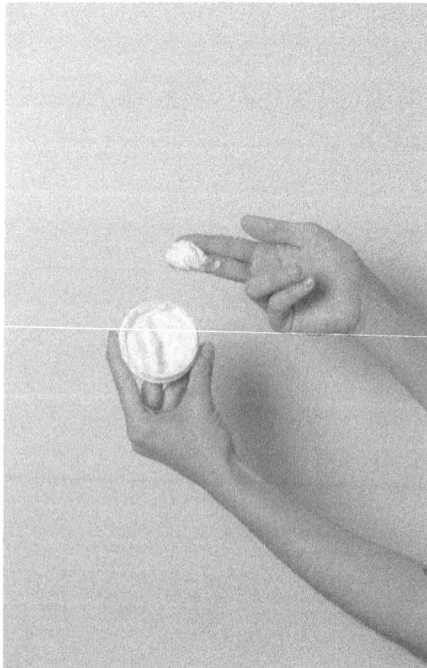

Inhibiting melanin production is a useful strategy to reduce spots, eventually eliminating their appearance. Depigmenting creams are used to treat dark spots and prevent new ones. The sun, advancing years, and hormones are the main reasons we turn to depigmenting creams. It should be noted that when using these creams, some lifestyle changes should occur. If your spots are caused by the sun, try to limit your sun exposure and use appropriate sunscreen.

Depigmenting creams typically contain Vitamin C, alpha hydroxy acids, Vitamin B3, serine, azelaic acid, and other lightening, active ingredients that work to reduce the appearance of stains (Nicolas, 2019). These ingredients provide some sun protection, but the use of an appropriate sunscreen is still advised.

Cream Application

Each product provides some guidelines regarding the proper use and application. Generally, a small amount of the product is applied to a clean and dry face. Don't treat depigmenting creams like a spot treatment. These products should be applied evenly over the entire face. Let the product sit for an hour before continuing your usual skincare routine.

You'll need to be patient and consistent with product application, as the effects are usually noticeable from six weeks onwards. Opt for depigmenting creams sold in pharmacies for the best quality. Below, I'll share some tips to help you get the best results out of your preferred product.

- *Apply at Night.* Depigmenting creams tend to be more effective at night. Always read the product label though, as some creams are suitable for daytime use.

- *Use Sunscreen.* Even if your preferred product has a built-in sunscreen, it is still advisable to use an appropriate sunscreen for your skin type. Oftentimes the SPF in depigmenting creams provides inadequate protection from the sun, so you can't rely on that alone.

- *Don't Overuse.* These treatments are designed to last a few weeks. If there is no noticeable improvement, then talk to a dermatologist.

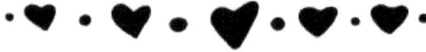

· ♥ · ♥ · ♥ · ♥ · ♥ ·

Oily Skin Cream

Oily skin presents a unique challenge. The secret to beautiful and hydrated skin lies in achieving balance. More specifically, a balance between excess sebum production and the natural moisture in the skin. Daily cleansing is essential to minimizing sebum on the face and maintaining the skin's pH levels. Exfoliants are a wonderful complement to any skincare routine. Regular use combats blackheads and evens skin texture. When cleansing the skin, it is important to massage the face with your fingertips. Doing so will ensure that oil and impurities are emulsified with the cleansing product, resulting in a deep and thorough clean.

A good product for oily skin will mattify the face. The hypoallergenic formulation should contain ingredients that won't clog the pores. Drinking water is a good, healthy habit to develop and is essential to prevent sebum overproduction. So don't hesitate to reach for that refreshing glass of water. Your skin will thank you!

Selecting a Cream

The hallmark of oily skin is excess sebum production. A regular moisturizing cream simply won't cut it. Gels are by far the best choice. These water-based products are easily absorbed and will not leave you with clogged pores.

Look at the label of products indicated for oily skin. These formulas should contain nourishing ingredients like Vitamin E, seaweed, and Vitamin C. These ingredients offer superior hydration without clogging the pores.

Finally, the product should offer some measure of sun protection to ward off sun damage and premature aging.

· ♥ · ♥ · ♥ · ♥ · ♥ ·

Anti-wrinkle Cream

You may be surprised to learn that anti-wrinkle creams do more than simply fight wrinkles. They play a role in repairing the dermis thanks to high concentrations of nourishing ingredients. On top of their repairing function, these creams typically have an exfoliating action to remove dead skin cells and improve the texture of the skin (Henríquez, 2018).

Many people opt to purchase non-prescription anti-wrinkle creams only to be disappointed by the results. The difference between over-the-counter creams and prescription creams is a simple, but very important one. Over-the-counter creams are not classified as a drug, therefore no scientific research is needed to prove their efficacy (Mayo Clinic, 2019). This means that all those skin-loving ingredients needed to combat fine lines are present in much lower concentrations in these products.

The efficacy of anti-wrinkle creams largely depends on the concentration of active ingredients. Popular ingredients in these products include retinoids, hydroxy acids, Vitamin C, Coenzyme Q10, peptides, tea extracts, grape seed extracts, and niacinamide. These ingredients are present in much lower concentrations in non-prescription creams. This means any results obtained are often short-lived. For the best results, search for an anti-wrinkle cream that contains these ingredients in relatively high concentrations. Anti-wrinkle creams need to be applied daily and consistently for noticeable results. If we discontinue usage of the product as soon as we see improvement, our skin is likely to return to its former appearance.

We also need to keep in mind that some products may cause side effects. If you experience any burning, rashes, or redness discontinue usage of the product and consult a dermatologist.

Maximizing Your Anti-wrinkle Regimen

It is no secret that the results of anti-wrinkle creams will vary with each product and individual. Fortunately, there are some steps you can take to enhance the results and get the most out of your anti-wrinkle regimen.

- *Sun Protection Is Vital.* Sun protection can be as simple as wearing a hat and sunscreen when you venture outside. Select products with built-in broadspectrum sunscreen for maximum protection.

- *Don't Forget to Moisturize.* Moisturizers boost our skin's water content and can temporarily improve the appearance of the skin.

- *Avoid Smoking.* Smoking narrows the blood vessels in our skin's outermost layers. Narrowed blood vessels mean fewer nutrients are reaching this part of the skin, damaging the collagen and elastin in the skin. This leads to premature wrinkles and sagging skin.

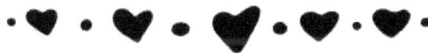

· ❤ · ❤ · ❤ · ❤ · ❤ ·

Nourishing Face Cream

There is a distinct difference between nourishing creams and moisturizers. Moisturizers help to increase the water content in the skin, while nourishing creams are designed to enrich the skin with lipids.

These creams help to nourish and regenerate the skin, providing vitamins, proteins, and lipids.

We use nourishing creams at night. These creams contain ingredients derived from Vitamins E and C, as well as other potent antioxidants. Sun exposure destroys the potency of these ingredients, rendering them ineffective. Apart from protecting ingredient integrity, another major reason we apply nourishing creams at night is that these creams function better when the face is relaxed. Sleep is a powerful ally and helps to activate these precious ingredients to trigger cell renewal and improve softness and elasticity.

Usage and Application

Nourishing creams (sometimes referred to as regenerating creams) should be used from the age of 30 onwards, although if you have particularly dry skin you can use them at an earlier stage. In our 30s, the cell renewal process starts to slow down, collagen and elastin break down quicker, and signs of life (wrinkles, bags under the eyes, and crow's feet) start to show up (Sinrich, 2018). Changing hormones also contribute to these changes. Nourishing creams gives the skin a helping hand by delaying signs of aging.

It is best to apply nourishing creams before you are ready for bed. After cleansing and toning the face, use a small amount and spread it evenly. Massage your face with your fingertips to ensure the product is fully absorbed into the skin.

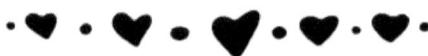

·❤ · ❤ · ❤ · ❤ · ❤ ·

Lip Balm

From delicious fruity flavors to playful pops of color, there is no shortage of variety when it comes to lip balm. These products are generally based on waxy formulas that are designed to protect the lips against cracking and drying. Lip balms weren't always the fruity medley we know and love—in the 19th century it was quite common to use earwax to protect the lips (TechnoReviews, 2019)!

Thankfully lip balms have evolved considerably since those early days and modern formulations often contain beeswax, cocoa butter, or carnauba. The lip balm market can be divided into three groups: balms containing sunscreen, colored balms, and moisturizing lip balms.

Balms containing sunscreen are recommended if you are planning any kind of prolonged sun exposure (like sunbathing, hiking, swimming, etc.). Colored lip balms are commonly used to replace lipsticks and can enhance the lips with a luscious pop of color. Moisturizing lip balms are best to use when we have dry lips or when the temperature drops to provide protection against cracking.

Before purchasing a lip balm, take a look at the packaging, fragrances, flavors, pigmentation, and solar protection that the product offers.

Most commonly, lip balm is presented in packaging quite similar to lipstick. This allows for easy application and transportation. Some balms are packaged in small pots, in which case you'll need to use a finger or applicator to apply.

Many lip balms have pigmentation and can be a handy alternative to lipstick. If you have allergies, it is best to opt for a basic lip balm that has no pigment, perfume, or flavor.

Our lips are quite sensitive and a lip balm with built-in UVA and UVB protection is handy to shield this delicate area against the sun's rays.

Regular usage of lip balms can help to prevent the lips from looking old. Yes, lips can age! Over time they become thinner and show small wrinkles. Keeping them nourished and hydrated can ensure that the signs of aging are delayed.

· ♥ · ♥ · ♥ · ♥ · ♥ ·

Sunscreen

Using the Fitzpatrick Scale to choose the correct SPF for your sunscreen is useful for adequate protection, however it can be tricky to know whether you should choose a cream, gel, spray, or stick. Below, you'll find tips that will help you select the correct sunscreen for your needs.

- Use creams for dry skin, gels on hairy areas, and sticks to protect the delicate eye area.

- Always opt for broad-spectrum sun protection whenever possible.

- If a sunscreen contains para-aminobenzoic acid (PABA or Vitamin Bx) don't use it. This organic compound is known to trigger allergic reactions.

- Sensitive skin will benefit the most from sunscreens that have titanium dioxide as the active ingredient (Cronan, n .d.).

Busting Sunscreen Myths

People who use broad-spectrum sunscreen daily age at a significantly slower rate than those who neglect applying the product. Regular use of sunscreen can reduce signs of aging by up to 24% (Scripps, 2013). With the significant role sunscreen plays to keep the skin youthful, it is surprising that some myths persist. Some of the most common myths include:

- ***Using Sunscreen Leads to Vitamin D Deficiency.*** There is no evidence to back this belief. The most likely source of vitamin deficiency is a poor diet. Many food sources such as salmon, eggs, and milk are rich in Vitamin D and should be included in a healthy eating plan.

- ***Sunscreen Is Not Needed When It's Cold or Cloudy.*** This is a very harmful myth that disregards the fact that up to 40% of UV radiation reaches the earth on a cloudy day. In addition to this, UV radiation can be reflected from many surfaces. Rather stay safe and use your sunscreen, even on overcast days. The sun's rays are strongest from 10 a.m. until 4 p.m., in the spring and summer.

- ***Most of Our Sun Exposure Comes from Childhood.*** This universal misunderstanding finds its roots in a study. The study found that we tend to get less than a quarter of our total sun exposure by the age of 18 (Skin Cancer Foundation, 2018). In reality, sun damage to the skin accumulates throughout life, and excessive exposure to sunlight can damage the skin's immune system. Sun damage accumulates and contributes to premature aging. Keep in mind that a sunburn develops over a 6 to 48-hour time span. It may be too late when you realize you've burned your skin.

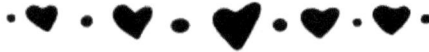

· ❤ · ❤ · ❤ · ❤ · ❤ ·

Masks

These products act quickly and are formulated with skin type in mind. They help to purify, hydrate, and illuminate the face. Before purchasing a face mask, there are two main things you need to consider.

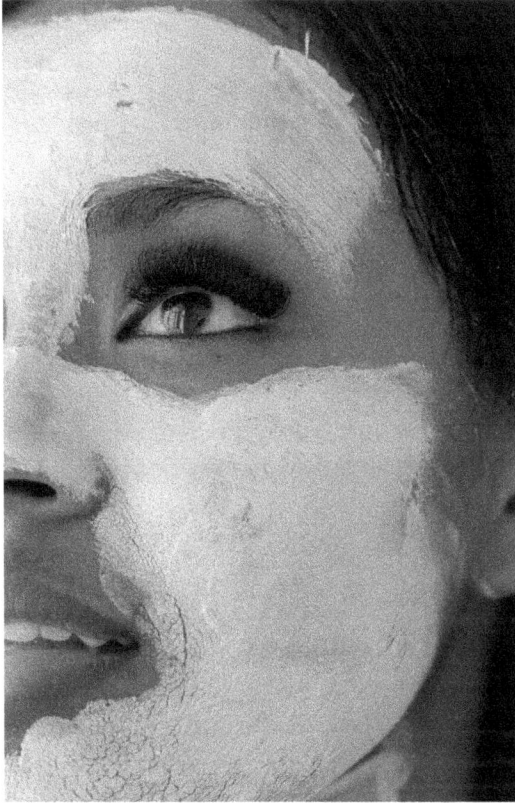

First, you'll need to select a product suited for your skin type. Dry skin will need a hydrating mask. Oily skin needs a mask that will absorb excess sebum and moisture. Soothing masks are the best option for sensitive skin.

Second, you'll need to consider when the mask will be used. Most masks are designed to be used at night to give the skin enough time to absorb all the nutrients present. However, some masks are meant to be used before we apply makeup.

All face masks aim to improve the appearance of the skin through hydration, exfoliation, and the absorption of excess fat. To this end, we find many different ingredients in masks including honey, lemon juice, oatmeal, egg yolk, clay, yogurt, cucumber, and coffee. Face masks can range from a gel to peel-off formulations, and each type is beneficial for a specific use.

- *Gel Masks:* Used to soften, tone, and refresh the skin. These masks help to lock moisture in the skin and are recommended for use on oily skin.

- *Powder Masks:* A clay or kaolin base absorbs excess oil from the skin and can assist with mild breakouts. These masks hydrate, soothe, and moisturize the skin.

- *Paste Facial Mask:* Commonly made by mixing water with clay, mineral salts, or algae. These masks are easy to apply and rich in antioxidants for a youthful, glowing appearance.

- *Solid Thermal Masks:* The main action of these masks is to increase the temperature of the face, triggering perspiration. These masks absorb excess sebum and can help to remove blackheads.

- *Organic Thermal Mud Mask:* A natural alternative to solid thermal masks.

- *Veil Masks:* Rich in collagen, these masks provide a powerful anti-wrinkle boost to the skin.

- *LED Facial Mask:* Through electrostimulation, these masks emit a series of light signals to treat a variety of skin problems.

- *Peel-off Mask:* These masks are applied to the face in a semi-liquid state. As the mask dries, it hardens and can be easily peeled off, making it ideal for facial cleansing.

Using Masks the Right Way

The use of facial masks improves the overall appearance of the skin and can lift your spirits by stimulating your senses. Unlocking all the benefits hidden in a face mask lies in the correct application.

- Cleanse your face. Combination and oily skin types will benefit from exfoliation. It helps the skin to optimally absorb the nourishing ingredients in the mask. Pat your face dry.

- Using the tips of your fingers apply the facial mask of your choice. Apply the product to your whole face, but avoid the sensitive lip and eye contour.

- Allow the mask to work its magic for 10 to 15 minutes. Some masks work faster, so always check the manufacturer's instructions for the correct time.

- When it is time to remove the mask, use lukewarm water. Use gentle, circular movement with your fingertips to "massage" the mask off. Keep in mind that your skin will be quite sensitive now, so you need to take every precaution not to irritate it.

- Lastly, apply moisturizer.

- Reapply the mask once (or twice) a week, but don't wait longer than 15 days between applications for best results.

Mask Mistakes

Using a mask as part of your regular skincare routine can have wonderful results if done the right way. To get the most out of your beauty routine, try to avoid these mistakes.

- *Applying the Mask to Unwashed Skin.* You should always wash your face before applying a mask, otherwise, all those good ingredients will be lost to dirt and bacteria. A great option is to cleanse the skin with micellar water to intensely purify the skin, allowing for maximum absorption of the mask's goodness.

- *Applying the Mask with Dirty Hands.* Clean hands are as important as a clean face. Unwashed hands can transfer oil and bacteria to the face, which can be counterproductive. For mess-free application use a flat foundation brush. Keep the brush aside and use it only to apply masks.

- *Using Too Much Product.* As with most things skincare, less is more. Applying a super-thick layer of the product will not give you better results, it will only waste the product. A single, even layer is enough.

- *Using Veil Masks As-Is.* Many times veil masks won't fit perfectly on the face, creating bubbles and leaving other areas uncovered. This problem can easily be solved with a pair of scissors, though. Snipp off any excess to ensure a better fit.

- **Using Masks Only While You Are Awake.** Some masks are formulated to be worn overnight, while others are meant to give your face a boost before applying makeup. Always check the manufacturer's instructions to make sure what the mask is intended for and when it should be used.

- **Leaving the Mask on Too Long.** If a mask is not indicated for overnight use, be mindful of the time! Leaving masks on for an extended amount of time does not mean you will get better results. Some ingredients can irritate when left on the skin for too long. Setting a timer is a useful strategy to avoid this problem.

- **Neglecting to Moisturize.** Masks provide an extra boost to the skin, but this does not mean the moisturizer should be ignored. If we ignore the moisturizing step, masking can result in dry and irritated skin (Evans, 2022).

- **Using a Single Mask.** Limiting yourself to a single mask may not be an effective strategy to address certain skin concerns. When we apply different masks to different areas of the face we can target certain concerns more effectively. This is a practice known as multi-masking. If you have combination skin you may want to apply a clay mask to the T-zone and a hydrating mask to your cheeks for a more customized result.

· ♥ · ♥ · ♥ · ♥ · ♥ ·

Care According to Skin Type

Your day and night routine most likely will follow the same basic steps of cleansing, toning, nourishing the skin, and hydrating. That being said, our skin has different care needs during the day and night. These needs are due to the skin's circadian rhythm. The skin becomes more permeable during the evening, making moisturizers and other topical treatments more effective (Lyons et al., 2019). These changes should be taken into account when considering your skincare. For this reason, certain products are formulated for day and nighttime use.

In the morning your skincare routine should focus on protection. As soon as you leave your home, your skin will be exposed to UV rays, pollution, and environmental factors. These variables can trigger oxidative stress, resulting in skin that feels thin, weak and unhealthy. It is always a good idea to include an antioxidant serum and moisturizer in your morning routine, followed by sunscreen. Opt for lightweight products if you plan on wearing makeup.

Your night routine should focus on cleansing and deeply nourishing the skin. Use the hardest working skincare products at night for maximum benefit. Keep in mind that the increased permeability of your skin during the night can lead to moisture loss, so don't skip your nourishing or regenerating cream.

Each face is different, so we will need to adopt a care routine that is suited for our specific skin type. Dry skin requires different care than oily or sensitive skin. When we use a skincare routine that is not suited for our skin type, we can encourage premature aging, trigger irritation, and cause blemishes to form.

Oily Skin Care Routine

Acne and breakouts are more likely to appear on oily skin due to excess oil accumulation. Your care routine should primarily focus on oil control to prevent future problems. These will be the steps to follow:

- Exfoliate once a week (twice if needed).

- Use a clay mask once a week.

- Cleanse the skin twice daily, followed by a toner and serum. Use the appropriate day and night products indicated for your skin type. Use gel formulations for effective, non-greasy skincare.

- Feed your skin with a nourishing gel.

- Finish the routine with sunscreen in the morning.

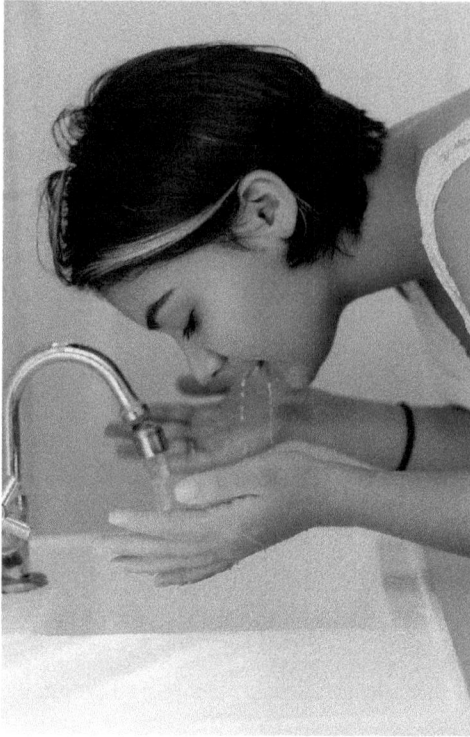

Dry Skin Care Routine

Caring for dry skin should center around maintaining maximum moisture in the skin. If this is your skin type, your routine will look something like this:

- Exfoliate and use a hydrating mask weekly.

- Cleanse and tone your skin in the morning.

- Apply a moisturizing serum followed by a moisturizing cream.

- Finish the routine with sunscreen.

- You may need to reapply moisturizer throughout the day if your skin is extremely dry.

- At night it is important to cleanse the skin using a milk, followed by a toner and serum. Finally, nourish your skin with a hydrating night cream.

Combination Skin Care Routine

The T-zone tends to become oily while the cheeks dry out. This makes combination skin a bit tricky and will require special care for each part of the face.

- Exfoliate weekly, followed by a mask. Use the multi-mask technique to control oil production in the T-zone, whilst hydrating and nourishing the cheeks.

- Cleanse twice daily. Use micellar water, followed by a toner to keep oil at bay.

- After cleansing, apply serum, followed by a moisturizing cream indicated for combination skin. Use a nourishing, revitalizing cream to complement your routine at night.

- Finish your routine with sunscreen in the morning.

Normal Skin Care Routine

This skin type is relatively easy to care for. Use products indicated for your skin type for optimal results. The skincare routine for normal skin types will look something like this:

- Exfoliate the skin weekly, followed by a mask.

- Cleanse the skin twice a day and apply toner.

- Apply serum and moisturize with the appropriate day or night cream.

- Finish your daytime routine with sunscreen.

Sensitive Skin Care Routine

Sensitive skin is prone to redness and irritation. Your skincare routine will need to balance, soothe, and hydrate the skin. Keep in mind that sensitive skin can be very reactive to new products, so try to keep your routine as simple as possible and avoid any harsh ingredients or fragrances.

- Gently exfoliate the skin weekly, followed by a mask. Select a mask with soothing and hydrating ingredients indicated for sensitive skin.

- Cleanse twice a day, followed by a toner.

- Apply a deeply hydrating serum after toning the skin.

- After the serum, apply a cream to lock in moisture. Focus on nourishing the skin at night.

- In the morning, apply sunscreen.

Now that the basics of good skin care are covered, you may want to learn how to treat blemishes and dark spots. In the next chapter, I'll shed some light on why Latina women struggle with dark spots and how they can be prevented and treated.

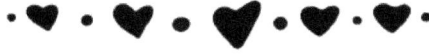

· ♥ · ♥ · ♥ · ♥ · ♥ ·

Four
Blemishes on the Face

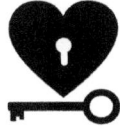

M arks and discoloration on the skin are commonly referred to as blemishes. Latin skin is particularly prone to produce more melanin, which can give rise to pigmentation alterations, i.e. blemishes (Robledo, 2021). In most cases, blemishes are harmless but we may wish to treat them for cosmetic reasons. It is natural to assign a much older age to someone with blemished skin than to an individual with even skin tone.

Different stains appear on the skin. Being able to differentiate between them and adjust your skincare routine accordingly is the key to successful outcomes. Blemishes can range from pink and red to white in color, but in most cases they are brown. Brown stains are linked to abnormal melanin production and most commonly appear on the face, hands, and neckline—our most sun-exposed body parts. These brown stains are referred to as hyperpigmented spots and can vary in size, shape, color, and origin. Moles, freckles, solar lentigines, and melasma are all examples of hyperpigmentation.

Types of Blemishes

Spots can appear through a combination of sun exposure, hormones, and hereditary factors. Freckles are typically hereditary and range from dark brown to yellow in color. Moles and solar lentigines (sun spots or age spots) form through the accumulation of melanocytes and melanin in the uppermost layers of the skin. They are typically not very large, but sun exposure can cause more to appear.

Other blemishes appear when melanin in a specific area increases. Sometimes the skin produces extra melanin after an injury or irritation. This is called post-inflammatory pigmentation (PIH). These marks tend to be flat and can vary from pink to grayish-brown in color and typically develop from acne marks and scars. When we have a wound, the body produces melanin as a response to cell damage, resulting in dark marks on the skin surface (Pond's, n.d.). Other times patches of pigmentation can develop due to hormonal changes or sun exposure, called melasma. Pregnant women are more likely to develop melasma and extensive cases can cover entire areas of the face.

Most blemishes appear on our skin during summer and autumn. During these months we tend to expose our skin to the sun for longer periods. Oftentimes this exposure goes hand in hand with inadequate sun protection. Fall is a time when most women will reach for depigmenting creams, which work quite well when stains are not deep in the skin.

·❤·❤·❤·❤·❤·

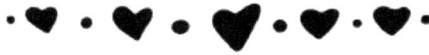

Preventing Blemishes

Skin has a memory. This means sun damage accumulates which can lead to spots appearing on the skin. Preventing blemishes is far easier than treating them and only requires a few small lifestyle changes.

- *Always Use Sunscreen.* Sunscreen should be applied before your skin is exposed to the sun. Most cases of premature aging, freckles, sun spots, and melasma are mainly caused by the sun. When we protect the skin with an appropriate SPF these problems are less likely to appear.

- *Cover Up.* Block out direct sunlight in addition to religiously using sunscreen. A simple, fashionable way to do this is by wearing a hat and sunglasses. Search for sunglasses that have UV protection and opt for a wide-brimmed hat to keep your face shaded.

- *Antioxidants Are Your Friend.* Skincare products with antioxidants as active ingredients are a good start, but you can't rely on them alone. Bolster your skincare regimen through a healthy diet rich in leafy greens, citrus fruits, berries, and foods containing Omega-3. Dietary sources of antioxidants help to reduce the damage done by free radicals and keep the skin healthy and glowing. Remember, your skin is essentially a cover letter for your health. Therefore, if your body is healthy, your skin will reflect it.

- ***Exfoliate and Brighten.*** There is no need to fret if the skin is already showing some signs of damage. Regular exfoliation and the use of a brightening serum can help to fade blemishes over time. If the spots are very dark, painful, and rough, see a dermatologist immediately.

- ***Nutriprotector for Fair Skinned Individuals.*** If you burn easily it may be in your best interest to use a nutriprotector. These capsules prepare the skin before sun exposure and can help to create a uniform and lasting tan (Farmacia Maiz Piat, 2019).

- ***Protect Your Scars.*** Scars should always be protected from the sun. The skin in these areas is more sensitive and tends to color easier.

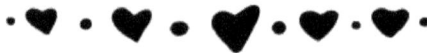

· ♥ · ♥ · ♥ · ♥ · ♥ ·

Effective Blemish Treatments

Over-the-counter treatment options for blemishes are usually centered around depigmenting creams. These products can be very effective as long as they are properly formulated. Key ingredients to look for are retinol and Vitamin C.

Retinol is effective in delaying the signs of aging and improves the appearance of expression lines. It can improve the appearance of dark spots for a beautifully even complexion. Retinol acts as a peeling agent and favors cell renewal, but we should take into account that not all retinoids are the same. Retinoic acid can only be obtained with a prescription, whereas other forms of retinol (retinaldehyde or retinil) are more commonly found on over-the-counter creams. Another thing we need to consider is the concentration of the active ingredients. The higher the concentration, the greater the efficacy, but it also increases the risk of irritation to the skin.

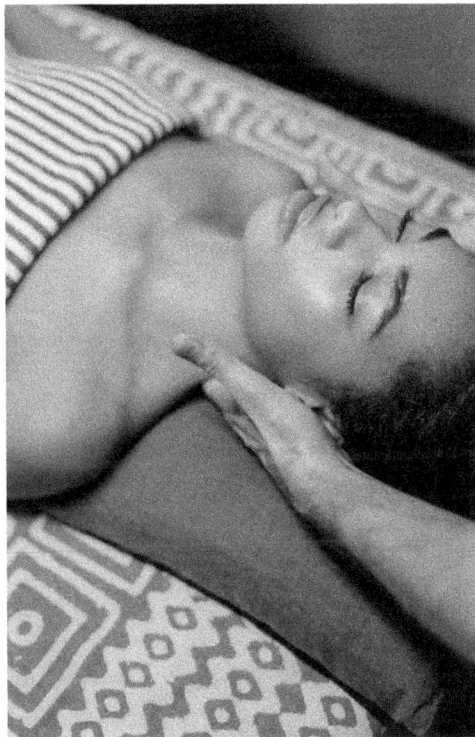

Vitamin C is another widely used ingredient to combat pigmentation spots. Continuous use has been shown to improve the appearance of the skin, brighten skin tone, and aid in restoring and calming the skin. This antioxidant works by protecting the skin from damage caused by free radicals and stimulates the production of collagen and elastin. For topical application, there are mainly two kinds that we can find. Pure Vitamin C (L-ascorbic acid) is the most effective, but also the most irritating to the skin. This form of Vitamin C is notoriously unstable and can lose its efficacy quickly if stored incorrectly. The stabilized version, ethyl ascorbic acid, is usually better tolerated on the skin, but is not as effective. In creams and serums, the ingredient is often identified as "ascorbic acid."

The treatment product you choose must come in an opaque container to protect the ingredients from sun and light exposure. Furthermore, these ingredients can oxidize and make the skin look "dirty," which is why a weekly exfoliant should accompany your treatment.

Brightening serums containing Vitamin C and niacinamide can be used together to soften the appearance of blemishes. These ingredients act through different mechanisms and complement each other, leaving your skin soft, supple, and less blemished with consistent use.

Over-the-counter treatments are most effective at reducing the prominence of recent and surface-level pigmentation stains. These treatments are not suitable for deeper stains.

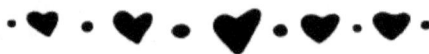

·❤ · ❤ · ❤ · ❤ · ❤ ·

Expert Stain Removal Options

A professional will be able to provide treatment for the most stubborn spots on the face. Depending on the diagnosis, the professional may suggest several options that include lasers, chemical peels, or oral treatment. Let's take a closer look at the treatment options your dermatologist could offer.

Hydroquinone

This is one of the most widely used treatments for dark marks (hyperpigmentation) on the face. Typically prescribed as a depigmenting cream, hydroquinone is often combined with kojic acid and retinoic acid to remove stains deep within the skin (Podlipnik, 2021). Retinoic acid is often used to treat blemishes and improve the appearance of wrinkles. Its oil-controlling properties make it a suitable ingredient in acne treatment as well.

Hydroquinone inhibits the production of melanin, which lightens blemishes over time. On average, visible results can be seen at week eight of treatment. This depigmenting cream is usually indicated for use on facial blemishes after pregnancy. While hydroquinone is generally safe to use, some people may experience dry skin, itching, and irritation as side effects. It is a good idea to perform a patch test before using hydroquinone creams, gels, or lotions. Simply apply a small amount of the product to your skin. Watch for signs of irritation—if the skin appears normal, it is safe to start treatment.

Laser Treatment

A far more aggressive option than the abovementioned cream, laser treatment can remove brown spots on the face through concentrated light energy. Some lasers target the pigment, while others remove the skin layer by layer. This treatment option is best reserved for age spots and chronic sun damage. Treatments are usually scheduled to be four to six weeks apart to give the skin enough time to heal.

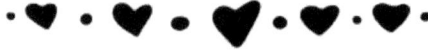

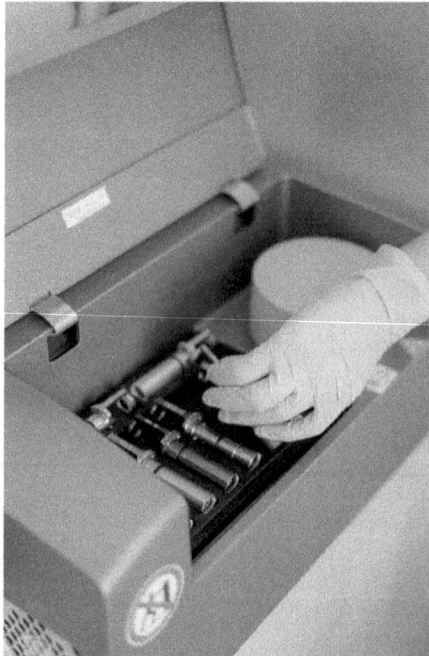

$\bullet\, \heartsuit \,\bullet\, \heartsuit \,\bullet\, \heartsuit \,\bullet\, \heartsuit \,\bullet\, \heartsuit \,\bullet$

Micro-Needling

When laser treatment is not an option (due to medical or other reasons) micro-needling comes into play. This minimally invasive treatment uses delicate titanium needles to stimulate the production of collagen in the skin. Micro-needling improves elasticity and is often used in combination with topical treatments. These treatments would contain tranexamic acid or Vitamin C, both of which have powerful effects on blemishes. Usually, a minimum of three treatments are required. These treatments are scheduled to be at least six weeks apart.

Chemical Peels

These treatments focus on removing the upper layers of the skin, stimulating collagen production over time, and reducing the appearance of dark spots. Typical active ingredients in chemical peels are glycolic, mandelic, salicylic, and lactic acid. Sessions are usually scheduled to be a month apart. Peels subscribe to one universal rule: the more powerful the peel, the fewer sessions you'll need. Of course with the increase in potency comes an increase in complications. Powerful peels are not recommended for sensitive skin and should only be done by a qualified person. There are many versions that you can use at home, but these peels usually don't penetrate the skin deep enough to make a difference in blemishes.

Oral Treatments

Tranexamic acid is an oral medication that inhibits melanin production. This medication is usually used in cases where the skin produces too much melanin, as is the case with melasma. Tranexamic acid is a second-line treatment and can be used during the summer when the usage of depigmenting creams is discontinued.

· ❤ · ❤ · ❤ · ❤ · ❤ ·

Home Remedies and Stain Removal

A quick internet search is enough to discover a wealth of "natural" and home remedies to remove dark marks. Many of these treatments may not have any proof and can have serious side effects. Common ingredients in these homebrews include lemon, baking soda, and apple cider vinegar. Sometimes these treatments can worsen spots and trigger dermatitis. Post-inflammatory hyperpigmentation (inflammation that darkens the skin) can cause the spots to worsen. Treatment can become difficult if the spots worsen beyond a certain point. Other harmful ingredients include corticosteroids and mercury. Application of remedies using these ingredients can lead to iatrogenic acne (acne caused by the treatment), facial rashes, and fragile skin. Simply put, it is not worth risking your beautiful face with a home remedy. Professionals are able to safely and effectively improve the appearances of blemishes. The results are longer lasting and guaranteed to be much gentler on the skin.

Five

Dark Circles in Latinas

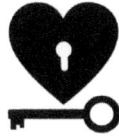

M any women have idiopathic orbital ring hyperchromia. You may know the condition under a more familiar name: dark circles. Dark circles can appear under the eyes even when the best skincare regimens are followed. Most of the time, it is assumed that the appearance of these unwelcome guests is due to a lack of sleep. The truth is that dark circles have many different causes. Tiredness, allergies, and aging all contribute to the appearance of dark circles.

The skin around the eyes is quite thin, making dark circles a fairly common problem. Common causes are changes in hormones, malnutrition, inadequate sun protection, smoking, the consumption of alcohol, and circulation problems. In addition to these common triggers, the eye contour has low levels of collagen. Water and toxins accumulate easily under the skin, giving a tired appearance to the face. Dark circles should not be confused with bags under the eyes. Although these problems are often twins, dark circles are characterized by an increase in pigmentation in the area. There are different kinds of dark circles, the color and appearance often give insight into the cause. The reference guide below will help you to speedily identify the root cause of dark circles.

- **Blue:** These are known as transient dark circles and are mainly caused by fatigue. They are the easiest to recognize. Tiredness, anxiety, and stress are common triggers for transient dark circles. Fortunately, they are easy to treat. Healthy lifestyle choices and getting enough sleep will help to keep these blue splotches away. Try to adjust your sleeping position, with your head slightly raised to discourage fluid accumulation around the eyes. Also, if you find yourself staring at the computer screen for most of the day, take regular breaks every 20 minutes to rest your eyes and ensure the screen is at least half a meter away from your eyes. A lack of iron is often associated with dark circles. Ensuring your diet contains enough iron is another step you can take to combat and prevent future dark circles. Red meat, leafy greens, citrus fruits, and egg yolk are rich sources of iron. If these circles are accompanied by bags under the eyes, it may be necessary to reduce your salt intake. A nutritionist can advise you if your diet is lacking in any essential nutrients.

- **Brown:** Hyperpigmented dark circles are caused by an increase in melanin production in the area and are normally genetic in origin. These are the most difficult to treat, and chances are, other family members will bear similar dark circles. Treatment often focuses on rebalancing hydration levels in the skin and providing firmness to the eye contour. A trained professional can advise you on the best treatment option.

- *Furrows:* These are caused by fat loss in the eye area and appear as marked furrows from the inner corner of the eye to the cheek. They are known as sunken dark circles and are mainly due to aging or health issues. Dehydration and vitamin deficiencies can contribute to the appearance of sunken eyes.

- *Purple or Dark Blue:* Vascular dark circles are caused by two things: dilation of the blood vessels and thinning of the skin in the eye area. Allergies are often the cause behind the appearance of these dark circles. When an allergy triggers the body, histamines are released into the bloodstream. Itchiness, redness, and puffy eyes are common symptoms, but histamines also dilate blood vessels, making them more visible beneath the skin (Cobb, 2022). In these cases, a cold compress may help to reduce puffiness and shrink dilated blood vessels. Alternatively, a compress with green tea or black tea may prove equally beneficial. Simply soak two tea bags in hot water for five minutes and place the bags in the fridge until cold. Pop the cold tea bags on your closed eyes for a few minutes to treat puffy eyes.

· ♥ · ♥ · ♥ · ♥ · ♥ ·

Preventing Dark Circles

The eyes accentuate your beauty. Dark circles can strip the face of that dewy, youthful look and assign one a much older appearance. It is only natural to resort to makeup to hide the appearance of dark circles, but doing so only masks the problem. Daily usage of makeup comes with one caveat: it can cause the deterioration process on your face if you don't clean it properly. The Dutch philosopher Desiderius Erasmus had it right all along when he stated that "prevention is better than cure." A few simple lifestyle adjustments are often enough to turn most dark circles into distant memory. However, some dark circles can persist even after reversible factors have been addressed. This is why pinpointing the root cause of your dark circles is important. If you are unsure what is causing your dark circles, a dermatologist can help.

- *Wear Sunglasses:* Protect your delicate eye area with sunglasses that have quality UV filters. The ideal would be to opt for a pair that offers protection against UVA and UVB rays. Don't forget to apply sunscreen before you leave the house.

- *Get Enough Sleep:* Most adults need seven to nine hours of quality sleep. To ensure your sleep is the best it can be, try to have a set bedtime routine. Avoid using any mobile devices before bedtime and try to hit the hay at the same time every night.

- *Eat a Balanced Diet:* When we eat healthily, this truth is reflected in our skin. Ensure your diet has enough Vitamin C, Vitamin K, zinc, and iron to prevent the appearance of nutrition-related dark circles. These nutrients are commonly found in broccoli, red pepper, lettuce, shellfish, nuts, and clams. A nutritionist can help you pinpoint which nutrients are lacking in your diet.

- *Cut Back on Coffee:* Ah, coffee! How would the modern world function without it? Excessive consumption of caffeine promotes all the things that can trigger dark circles to appear, though: anxiety, restlessness, and trouble sleeping (Petre, 2020). Cutting back on those caffeinated brews can go a long way to help reduce the appearance of dark circles.

- *Stay Hydrated:* Our bodies need to remain hydrated to allow proper blood circulation and functioning. If any problems with circulation occur, it is usually reflected in the blood vessels. Avoiding dehydration is one of the simplest steps you can take to prevent dark circles and give your skin a boost. Don't wait until you are thirsty to drink water, reach for that refreshing glass of H2O regularly throughout the day. Aim to drink two liters of water a day. Your skin and body will thank you.

- *Use Eye Contour:* These products are specially formulated to treat the delicate eye area without irritation. Slapping on any ol' moisturizer will not do the trick and may promote premature aging in the eye area. To treat dark circles, opt for an eye contour that deeply moisturizes and treats irregular pigmentation. Apply the eye contour with a light massage to promote better product absorption and functioning.

- *Exercise:* Regular exercise is important to encourage circulation and can help with the elimination of fluid retention. Exercise is also a useful tool to get rid of stress, which can lead to better sleep and the reduced appearance of dark circles.

- *Get Those Allergies Treated:* Taking the appropriate medication and staying away from possible allergy triggers will help to keep this immune reaction under control. Avoid rubbing your eyes when they itch, as the blood vessels in the area are very delicate and can easily be damaged.

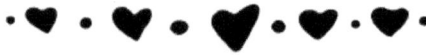

· ♥ · ♥ · ♥ · ♥ · ♥ ·

Effective Treatments for Dark Circles

Dark circles, even the tricky hereditary ones, don't have to be a life sentence! With advances in treatment technology, there are many options available for women who wish to reduce the appearance of these gremlins. Treatments in a professional setting can range from non-invasive treatments, like peels and laser treatments, to surgical options. In this section, we will explore all the different professional and home-based treatment options available.

Professional Treatment Options

The color of dark circles will often dictate the treatment plan that is recommended. Some of the most recommended treatments in the professional setting include periorbital rejuvenation, carboxytherapy, peeling, laser treatment, and blepharoplasty. Let's take a look at what each of these procedures entails.

- *Periorbital Rejuvenation:* This treatment option does not require allergy testing before application, because it makes use of hyaluronic acid. These microfilaments are injected at strategic points to rejuvenate the eye contour. Results are usually most noticeable at the three-week mark. The effects of hyaluronic acid can last up to two years.

- *Carboxytherapy:* Carbon dioxide is used in this treatment technique to counter the effects fatigue, stress, and genetic factors can have on the appearance of dark circles. Carboxytherapy uses the lymphatic system to improve skin tone and eliminate toxins.

- *Peeling:* During the peeling procedure, material is layered on the dark circles and then neutralized to achieve a depigmenting effect. It is normal to feel a little tightness in the lower eye area after the procedure, but your skin will become fresher and smoother in the days that follow.

- *Laser Therapy:* Laser treatment falls into two categories, vascular laser, and depigmentation laser treatment. Vascular laser treatment is used to close visible blood vessels, reducing the appearance of dark purple dark circles. Blood vessels are cauterized through heat and it is a painless effective treatment option. Sessions are scheduled a month apart and are often complemented with orbital rejuvenation. Laser treatments are used to get rid of excess melanin caused by sun exposure and hormonal changes, both of which play a role in the appearance of blemishes. On average, six sessions are needed. Each session is scheduled to be two weeks apart, to improve the appearance of dark brown circles under the eyes.

- *Blepharoplasty:* This treatment option requires you to go under the knife. It is used to treat eye bags that appear due to congenital factors. This type of surgery should not be confused with an "eye lift." It does not raise eyebrows or eliminate circulatory dark circles. The technique is purely used to remove excess skin from the lower part of the eye.

- *Fibroblast Therapy:* Non-surgical treatment that lifts and tightens the skin around the eye. Using a plasma pen, the professional stimulates collagen production to rejuvenate the eye area, getting rid of bags, dark circles, and fine lines. Sagging and wrinkles on the upper eyelid can also be improved with surprisingly quick results. The procedure takes 30 to 60 minutes to complete and results are seen instantly. Best results can be seen after three to six treatments. Usually, one to three treatments at six-week intervals are recommended to obtain results comparable to a surgical procedure.

Home Treatments

Creams and serums formulated for the eye area are some of the go-to treatment options many women reach for. When selecting creams and serums the ingredients are vital. Look for these ingredients on the label:

- **_Retinol:_** With repeated use retinol can help to stimulate collagen production. This treatment route is especially recommended when dark circles are caused by the thinning of the skin and can help to recover skin volume and firmness.

- **_Vitamin C And Kojic Acid:_** When dark circles are caused by increased pigment production, it is best to opt for serums and eye contour that contain lightening ingredients. Vitamin C and kojic acid help to decrease skin pigmentation with consistent use. To prevent future darkening of the skin, use a broad-spectrum sunscreen that contains zinc oxide. Sometimes titanium oxide is used instead.

- **_Caffeine:_** While drinking too much caffeine can lead to dark circles, topical application of caffeine can be beneficial for treating puffy, tired eyes and purple dark circles. Caffeine is an ingredient found in many creams designed to reduce the appearance of tired and puffy eyes. These products work because caffeine is a vasoconstrictor. It tightens blood vessels temporarily to reduce the appearance of dark circles and can reduce redness, swelling and fluid retention.

Dark circles usually don't indicate a medical problem, but if you find you have discoloration under one eye that worsens over time it is best to seek medical advice. At-home treatments can successfully be used to treat mild dark circles. To treat trickier dark circles it is best to employ professional help. Apart from dark circles, we often seek professional help with another familiar skin problem: acne. In the next chapter, we take a deeper look into the causes of adult acne and the steps you can take to reclaim your glorious skin.

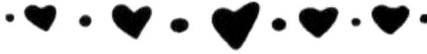

· ♥ · ♥ · ♥ · ♥ · ♥ ·

Six

Acne in Latin Adult Women

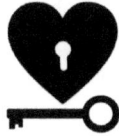

A cne does not end during the teenage years. For many women, the struggle with acne continues well into their twenties. Roughly 12% of women after the age of 25 find themselves seeking help for adult acne (Rivera & Guerra, 2009). Men and women older than 45 are less likely to struggle with this problem.

Women with adult acne tend to naturally produce more sebum than women who don't. Cosmetics, drugs, our environment, and stress also play a role in the prevalence of acne. If you are a smoker between the ages of 25 and 50, I've got some bad news. You are roughly 40% more likely to develop acne than your non-smoking counterparts (Schafer et al., 2001). The prevalence of acne in smokers is higher because tobacco triggers the development of acne in pre-disposed people. Smoking encourages the small veins in our skin to narrow, influencing the blood supply and nutrients our skin receives.

The risk of adult acne increases if you have first-degree relatives who've suffered from the condition. Nearly half of adult acne cases can be linked to family history (Goulden et al., 1997).

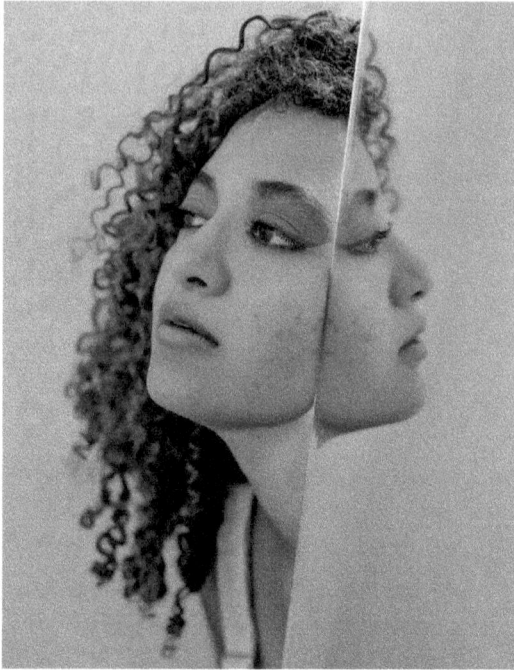

Many adult acne cases can also be linked to women who experience abnormalities during the menstrual cycle. In a minority of patients, adult acne can indicate the presence of Polycystic Ovary Syndrome (PCOS). This syndrome is characterized by an irregular cycle, increased body hair, and weight gain. It is always advisable to rule out PCOS first when dealing with adult acne. Visiting a medical professional will rule out any hormonal abnormalities. Acne in adult women has also been linked to the overuse of cosmetics, peels, and masks (Guarino, 2021).

Other acne triggers include excessive sun exposure, diet, sleep disturbances, excessive face washing, and using the wrong skin care products for your skin type.

Acne at any age can significantly impact our quality of life, confidence, relationships, and daily activities. The impact goes deeper than simply feeling self-conscious when going out for the evening. Studies found that the psychological impact acne has is on par with diabetes, epilepsy, and arthritis (Ramos-e-Silva et al., 2015).

Acne can be quite resistant to treatment and can be classified as persistent or late-onset acne in some cases. If acne was present since adolescence it is generally classified as persistent acne. These are characterized by lesions and can worsen during the menstrual cycle. The lesions (also called epidermal inclusion cysts) are solitary, slow-growing and vary in size. The face, scalp, and neck are popular places for these uninvited guests to appear.

Late-onset acne only appears after puberty. This form of acne is usually subdivided into two categories: inflammatory acne and sporadic acne. Inflammatory acne tends to affect women who suffer from premenstrual exacerbations. These women typically experience worsened anxiety, increased irritability, mood swings, and fatigue before the onset of their cycle. Unfortunately, this type of acne is quite resistant to treatment and can produce scarring and pigmentation marks. Sporadic acne can be seen in adults over 60. There appears to be no reason for the appearance of this type of acne and it mainly affects the chest area.

· ♥ · ♥ · ♥ · ♥ · ♥ ·

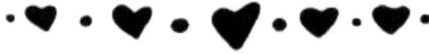

Acne-Forming Habits

Many of our habits give acne a foothold in our lives. We don't give stress the habit-forming credit that it is due (Schwabe & Wolf, 2009). When we have high-stress levels, the production of certain hormones (like androgens, cortisol, and adrenaline) increases. The result shows up on our faces in the form of acne. Stress is hardly the only bad habit that encourages acne. To help you identify these habits ask yourself:

- *Am I Drinking Enough Water?*

It is possible that you are not. Shockingly, nearly 40% of Hispanic adults do not drink enough water (Brooks et al., 2017). Water functions a bit like a washing machine, cleaning toxins from the body. If we don't drink enough water, the results will show up on the skin in the form of acne, dullness, wrinkles, and loss of firmness.

- *Am I Using the Correct Products Correctly?*

When we use cleanser willy-nilly, skip the toner, or use a moisturizer for a different skin type, acne is often the result. Furthermore, facial products that are very alkaline can damage the skin, as we discovered in chapter three. It is only logical to reach for topical acne treatments when we spot those unwelcome guests, but incorrect use can cause more acne as a result. Other products containing alcohol can dry out the skin. This makes it easier for bacteria to breach our skin's defenses. So taking a good, hard look at your skincare products and their ingredients is an important first step to an acne-free future.

- ### *Do I Have a Healthy Diet?*

There are two culprits you need to look out for: hormones and sugar. Dairy and other fatty foods may contain hormones that can directly affect the body's hormone levels, resulting in adult acne. Limit your intake of these foods and shop for clean foods, i.e., free-range, hormone-free, antibiotic-free products, and non-processed foods whenever possible. Another consideration is the amount of sugar in a diet. High sugar levels stimulate the production of androgens, which leads to acne (Sanchez, 2019).

- ### *Am I Drinking Too Much Alcohol?*

Excessive alcohol consumption hits the body with a quick one-two jab. First, it dilates blood vessels and dehydrates the body, making it easier for bacteria to invade the skin. Second, it adds a lot of sugar to our diets. Many alcoholic beverages (cocktails especially) are high in sugar, which in turn messes with certain hormones. It is a vicious cycle, but it can be broken!

Not All Bumps Are Acne

Other skin conditions such as acne rosacea and perioral dermatitis are often mistaken for acne. There is a critical difference though as these conditions tend to appear in middle-aged women who have sensitive skin, whereas adult acne is indiscriminate of skin type.

Corticosteroids and many other medications can trigger acne-like eruptions on the face and upper body. Infection of hair follicles and damp, hot conditions can trigger acne-like breakouts on the skin.

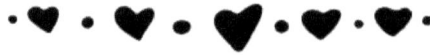

• ♥ • ♥ • ♥ • ♥ • ♥ •

Preventing Acne

Stay those fingers! Declare war on acne, but do it the right way. While it may be tempting, popping zits is not the right way to do it. When pimples burst (especially if we give them a helping hand) it is an open invitation for bacteria to infect the skin (Sherry, 2022). This gives us a whole new problem to deal with—scars. In this section, I'll share many valuable tips you can follow to prevent this problem in the future.

- *Give Your Skin a Break.* Limit your makeup use. While we can easily hide pimples with makeup, it is not recommended. This practice only encourages more pimples to appear. There are cosmetics with acne-treating properties, but you should not rely on them alone.

- *Get Moving.* A healthy lifestyle will always encourage

beautiful skin. As we work up a sweat, our bodies expel toxins. In the long run, this means fewer breakouts.

- *Learn to Relax*. Stress can wreak havoc on our hormones, the results often reflecting on our skin. Take some time to relax each day to offset those daily stresses. Your hormones and skin will thank you.

- *Learn to Love Omega-3.* Fruits, vegetables, salmon, and nuts are rich in omega-3 and can easily be added to your diet. Omega-3 is anti-inflammatory, and since acne is associated with inflammation, these fatty acids may be helpful (Streit, 2021). It is best to see a dermatologist if you find your acne worsens.

- *Stay Hydrated and Clean.* Following a structured face care routine (like the skincare routines in chapter three) is vital for beautiful skin. These routines will help you remove impurities and replenish moisture. This level of care is needed to prevent breakouts and speed recovery along.

- *Care for Your Hair and Scalp.* Our hair can trap a surprising amount of oil and dirt which can be transferred to the skin, especially when it hangs over the face. Keeping the hair clean and out of the face will go a long way in preventing future outbreaks.

· ♥ · ♥ · ♥ · ♥ · ♥ ·

Preventing Acne Marks

An important rule of thumb to remember with acne is this: the greater the swelling, the bigger the possibility of scarring (Press, 2018). For Latinas, prevention becomes even more important! Darker skin tones tend to form keloids and hypertrophic scars more frequently, which can be tricky to treat. Save yourself future troubles by following these tips.

- *Leave Them Alone.* Don't pick. Don't squeeze. A fairly simple step, but one that can reduce the occurrence of acne scars significantly. When we pick and squeeze acne, we injure our skin and encourage scar tissue to develop. Manipulating acne and damaging the skin can lead to scarring—more on that later.

- *Don't Ignore the Severity.* A topical treatment used for mild breakouts will not be effective against severe breakouts. These require a different treatment route and possibly help from a professional. Dermatologists, cosmiatrists, and dermocosmiatrists all complement each other and can be approached for help. Early and correct treatment is vital if we want to avoid scars.

- *Superficial Acne Marks Will Vanish.* It takes about a year for shallow acne scars to disappear, but the process can be sped up with peelings, micro-needling, and serums rich in retinol. Deeper scars will require a different treatment route, which I'll cover in a moment.

- *Listen to the Professional.* If you visit a professional for help, follow their instructions closely and use the products as advised for best results.

Options for Deep Acne Scars

For deeper acne scars that are older than a year, several treatment options are available. Any professional worth their salt will tell you that these treatments should only be applied after the inflammatory stage (active pimple stage) of acne has passed. They will recommend a suitable treatment plan.

Moderate to severe breakouts can form scar tissue that leaves the skin discolored and filled with indentations. These scars usually don't improve over time. Your dermatologist may recommend a bleaching cream and sunscreen to address the problem. There are several options for indentations in the skin.

- *Laser Skin Repair:* Also called laser resurfacing, helps to improve skin tone and appearance by stimulating collagen production.

- *Intense Pulsed Light (IPL):* This treatment makes use of pulsed light sources and radiofrequency devices to make scarring less noticeable.

- *Injectables:* In some cases the skincare professional may choose to inject soft tissue fillers or botulinum toxin (Botox) to treat scarring and reduce puckering (Hand, 2017). The treatment option depends on the nature of the scars.

- *Chemical Peels and Thermal Abrasion:* For severe cases of scarring, a dermatologist may recommend chemical peels or thermal ablation as treatment routes. These procedures can help reduce the appearance of deeper scars but require a longer recovery time.

- *Surgery.* Think of this procedure as a mini skin graft. Keep in mind the emphasis is on 'mini' here. It is a minor procedure where acne scars are removed one by one. You'll receive care instructions to help the skin heal as beautifully as possible. Another procedure involves inserting needles under the skin to improve scar appearance. This is called subcision. Each procedure comes with its own benefits and potential for side effects.

Reducing acne scars may require a combination of treatments. It is always best to consult with your dermatologist for the best solution. The highest prevalence is seen in the African population, followed by the Asian and Hispanic populations, and less frequently in Caucasians.

Hypertrophic and Keloid Scars

Every Latina needs to know this: the highest prevalence of hypertrophic and keloid scars are seen in people of African, Asian, and Hispanic descent (Carswell & Borger, 2020). Acne scars heal in different ways. Sometimes they do not extend beyond the original injury site, which would be a hypertrophic scar (Gauglitz et al., 2011). If that same acne scar heals differently and projects beyond the original wound margins, you've got a keloid scar. Your dermatologist can offer you a variety of treatment options.

- *Surgery.* Your dermatologist will recommend the appropriate procedure when applicable.

- *Silicones.* The use of silicones has become widespread since the 80s. This treatment is available in gel or sheets to reduce the appearance of scars. It is often used in combination with other treatments.

- *Compression.* This treatment approach applies pressure on the scar tissue, over time improving the appearance.

- *Corticosteroids.* The topical use of corticosteroids can improve the appearance of scar tissue and is often used as a second-line option for hypertrophic scars (Andrades et al., 2006). As with any treatment option, there are pros and side effects that a dermatologist will explain.

- ***Cryotherapy and Laser.*** Just so you know, cryotherapy hurts and involves freezing the scar. A similar method is used to remove moles sometimes. Laser therapy may be a suitable alternative as well. Your skin care professional will always recommend the best option.

Therapies can be used in isolation, but are oftentimes combined for best results. If any of these treatment options apply, the skin care professional will provide you with a care plan and instructions. These should be closely adhered to for an optimal outcome.

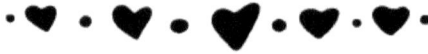

· ♥ · ♥ · ♥ · ♥ · ♥ ·

Treatment Options

Professionals can distinguish the severity of acne quite easily. They evaluate the types of lesions and other important factors to inform their treatment recommendation. If you tried non-prescription acne products to no avail, it is high time to find help.

Acne medications work on three levels. They reduce oil production, treat bacterial infection and improve swelling. Your age, severity, and type of acne and commitment to the treatment will ultimately determine which treatment plan is best. Treatment options include topical medications, oral medications, and therapies.

Topical Medications

Moderate cases of acne are sometimes treated with retinoic acids. These treatments can come in cream, gel, and lotion formulations for easy application. Typically we would apply this medication every third night for the first week. This application method reduces the risk of skin irritation. After a week we can apply the treatment daily. Retinoic acid is a photosensitizer, that is, during treatment it must be protected from the sun.

On other occasions, a professional may recommend antibiotics. Antibiotics target bacteria and help to reduce redness and the associated swelling. This treatment route can be quite long depending on the severity of the problem. The topical application of benzoyl peroxide usually complements this treatment option for optimal results. If antibiotics fail, antiandrogen agents may be prescribed. These medications work by blocking the effect of androgen hormones, thereby preventing breakouts. As a last resort, isotretinoin (a derivative of Vitamin A) is prescribed. This option is usually reserved when other treatment routes did not improve the appearance of severe acne.

There is insufficient evidence to support the efficacy of zinc, sulfur, aluminum chloride, nicotinamide, sodium sulfacetamide, and resorcinol in topical acne treatments (Mayo Clinic, n.d.).

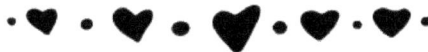

· ♥ · ♥ · ♥ · ♥ · ♥ ·

Therapies

Each individual is different. For some people, phototherapy and chemical exfoliation work well. In other cases, a professional may need to use special tools to remove impurities. Acne should be treated as soon as possible to reduce and prevent the possibility of scarring and discoloration.

Home Treatment Approach

Your daily skincare routine will likely need a little tweaking during a breakout. Use a mild non-drying cleanser. A cleanser containing salicylic acid or benzoyl is a good option if the skin is acne-prone. Make sure to remove all makeup and dirt. Double cleanse with micellar water at night. Micellar water effortlessly attracts dirt and grease, clears pores, and tones skin (Link, 2020). Complete your skincare routine as you normally would and apply a topical spot treatment. It is best to use products that are water-based and non-comedogenic.

A few lifestyle changes can lend a big hand in the battle against acne. Pin your hair out of your face and avoid oil-based cosmetics. Avoid tanning booths and excessive sun exposure. Your skin may become a bit more sensitive with acne treatment. It's temporary, but you'll need to take extra care of your skin during that time. Avoid foods that seem to make your acne worse (MedLine Plus, n.d.-a). The last adjustment you would need to make is to avoid tight headbands, hats, and baseball caps for the time being. These small adjustments help to speed up recovery time.

Ice can be a nifty ally to reduce inflammation when acne catches you off guard. Place a wrapped ice cube on the affected area to reduce swelling. Never place naked ice against your skin, as it can be damaging. The efficacy will depend on the severity of the breakout.

If you need to disguise blemishes, use a creamy concealer for better coverage. Powder and liquid concealers can draw attention to the blemish (L'Oreal Paris, n.d.). Use products formulated for acne-prone skin. Acne is not the only affliction that can plague the skin. Atopic dermatitis is estimated to affect 10% of the global population (Eucerin, n.d.-a). I'll dive deeper into this topic in the next chapter.

· ♥ · ♥ · ♥ · ♥ · ♥ ·

Seven

Atopic Dermatitis

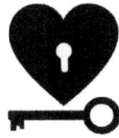

Atopic dermatitis (AD) is a fairly common inflammatory disease that affects 30 million Americans (Cantu-Pawlik, 2019). Latinos and children are among the most vulnerable groups to be affected by AD. Genetics and the environment play a leading role here. Atopic dermatitis usually starts during infancy and early childhood but can develop in adulthood as well.

We normally observe cases of atopic dermatitis where family history is present or if other conditions (asthma and allergies) are present. Genetics should not be ignored, as it determines the functioning of skin barrier cells and skin immune cells. Certain mutations can impact the functioning of these skin cells, which may help to explain why certain individuals and ethnic groups are more at risk of developing AD.

What many people fail to understand is that AD looks different on darker skin tones. The condition is often described as a red, dry, and itchy rash—and this description holds true... for light skin tones. In darker skin tones, redness may be difficult to see, and flare-ups can look dark brown, purple, or ash gray (Kaufman & Alexis, 2018).

With the characteristic red missing, it can be easy to dismiss those itchy patches as something else.

In people of color, some unique forms of AD may arise. In dark skin tones, small bumps could form on the torso, legs, and arms. This is known as papular eczema. Sometimes these bumps develop around hair follicles. In rare cases, prurigo nodules can develop. The exact cause of the condition is not understood, but it's believed that frequent scratching and picking triggers the condition to develop [NORD (National Organization for Rare Disorders), n.d.]. It is quite rare though and you'll need to be diagnosed by a professional.

Another challenge atopic dermatitis presents in darker-skinned women is uneven skin tone. The skin may be left with an uneven color when AD improves. This can be particularly bothersome on the face. The skin tone does even out, but it takes a long time. With the help of skin care professionals, this problem can be successfully resolved.

•❤•❤•❤•❤•❤•

Spot the Symptoms

AD often flares up in the face. The information in this section will help you recognize the symptoms and determine possible causes. The symptoms may vary, depending on the location of the body. We'll only focus on the symptoms of this condition in the face.

- The skin is dry and irritated, prone to flaking, cracking, and thickening.

- The affected area can become intensely itchy, red, and inflamed.

- Skin rashes may develop.

- Sunlight may or may not be a trigger. In some people sunlight eases symptoms, while others find it a trigger (Eucerin, n.d.-a).

Symptoms can vary between people, seasons, and days, but the distinct phases of AD are pretty consistent. There is the acute phase (also called a flare-up). The skin is the itchiest and most irritable during this stage. This phase is followed by a calmer period. Triggers play a role in flare-ups and vary from person to person, but can include:

- Climate

- Pollution

- Stress

- Harsh facial cleansers

- Inappropriate makeup products

- Allergens (wool, detergents, etc.)

The symptoms should be treated like triggers. The first instinct we have when we feel an itch is to scratch. When we scratch, bacteria can infect the skin and cause inflammation and more itching. The worsened itching leads to more scratching and more itching. We call this the Atopic Skin Cycle.

AD does not have a cure at this stage, but with the rate skincare science is advancing, there is hope. The condition can be managed, but there are a few steps you'll need to take to limit flare-ups and triggers as much as possible.

- *Moisturize Regularly*

The main goal when treating atopic dermatitis is to prolong the non-active phase. This is where regular moisturization is vital. Carefully evaluate the ingredients on the label. Look for proven ingredients to soothe, strengthen, and nourish the skin. Licochalcone A, ceramides, and omega-3 are often used.

- *Cleanse Gently*

Harsh cleansers and hot water will irritate the skin. Use a mild cleanser and avoid temperature extremes when rinsing with water. Water that is too hot can dry the skin more.

- *Shield Your Face from the Sun*

Always protect your skin by using products that are suitable for your skin type. This simple step can prevent a lot of future skin damage.

- ### *Choose Cosmetics Wisely*

Fragrance-free products formulated for sensitive skin are good options when needed. Be sure to remove all traces of makeup at night.

- ### *Unwind*

Stress is one of the most significant triggers and can make AD worse (Bard, 2021). Stress increases inflammation, which could explain why it can worsen the condition.

- ### *Keep an Eye on Weather Apps and Forecasts*

Extreme changes in temperature and certain weather conditions can act as triggers in some people. Knowing what the weather is up to will help you take preventative steps, limiting the impact.

$$\cdot \heartsuit \cdot \heartsuit \cdot \heartsuit \cdot \heartsuit \cdot \heartsuit \cdot$$

The Personal Impact

AD can have an impact on one's emotional and mental wellbeing. We may feel self-aware, ashamed, embarrassed, or frustrated because the condition takes time and effort to manage. Research has found that people with AD are more likely to be diagnosed with depression than those without the condition (Kowalczyk, 2020). It is not surprising, though. Some people with AD may feel more inclined to self-isolate during flare-ups. Other people experience increased levels of stress and anxiety, which could trigger more flare-ups. Some lifestyle interventions may be necessary to successfully manage the condition. These mainly focus on reducing stress levels in various ways.

- **Breathing Exercises:** Deep breathing methods found in yoga can promote relaxation and ease stress and anxiety symptoms.

- **Meditation:** Meditation turns into an effective stress-buster by promoting a sense of calm. In the long run, it can lower stress levels to help manage AD symptoms and reduce flare ups.

- **Get Enough Sleep:** Sleep is essential to reducing the levels of stress hormones in the bloodstream.

- **Watch Funny Cat Videos:** It may sound like odd advice, but there's a method to the madness. Watching those funny cat videos can help to lower stress (Kowalczyk, 2020). That's because laughter can improve mood and our immune system's functioning.

- **Reach Out:** I'll tweak a famous quote from T.A. Webb a little here. A journey shared is a burden halved. Some people share their experiences and tips for managing AD in support groups.

Treating Atopic Dermatitis

Treating atopic dermatitis will depend on the causes and symptoms. A skincare professional will recommend the correct treatment. Some useful tips can offer relief:

- *Use Anti-inflammatory and Antipruritic Products.* Hydrocortisone cream may temporarily reduce symptoms and oral antihistamines can reduce itching. A professional may recommend these to complement the treatment plan.

- *Check the Label.* Applying a moisturizer while the skin is still damp can help to improve symptoms. Check the label for 12% ammonium lactate or 10% alpha hydroxy acid for relief from dry, flaky skin (Mayo Clinic, n.d.-b).

- *Use Medicated Shampoos.* Shampoos containing coal tar, selenium sulfide, and pyrithione zinc can help control dandruff.

- *Soften the Scratch.* Wear gloves while you sleep and keep the nails short to reduce skin damage done by scratching.

- *Avoid Known Triggers.* It is a non-negotiable step in the journey to managing AD. Triggers will vary in each case.

- *Choose Cotton.* It is recommended to stay away from wool, plastic, rubber, and synthetic fibers where possible, as these may irritate the skin (Sendagorta Cudós & de Lucas Laguna, 2009).

Eight
Top 23 Supplements to Rejuvenate Your Face

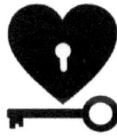

A s we age, our skin undergoes interesting changes, and your skincare routine will need to take these changes into account. The epidermis thins and the number of melanocytes decreases, giving the skin a pale appearance in some cases. Pigmented spots may appear in sun-exposed areas.

The skin becomes weaker and loses its elasticity through the aging process. Women produce less oil as they advance in years, resulting in dry and itchy skin (MedLine Plus, n.d.-b). Blemishes crop up more frequently due to the fragile nature of the skin.

Maintaining skin health can have a significant impact on how gracefully we age. Where skincare is concerned, there are two types of aging: photoaging and chronological aging. Photoaging is a result of accumulated sun damage. Chronological aging is the natural aging process. In the greater scheme of things, proper skin care and supplementation can help us delay the signs of aging significantly.

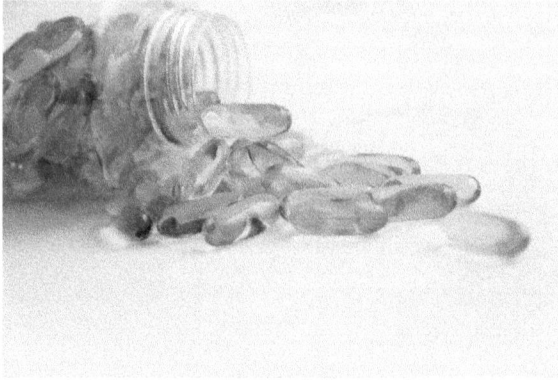

Vitamins are essential for the proper functioning of our bodies. Regular intake of vitamins through a healthy diet or supplementation will encourage smooth, hydrated, and healthy skin. It also promotes the formation of collagen and elastin for firmer skin. Young skin is characterized by its firmness, elasticity, and moisture retention abilities, and vitamins help to support these abilities optimally.

There are times when the skin will reveal that it needs nourishment. If you experience pale, loose, dry, cracked, wrinkled, or spotty skin it may be a sign of undernourishment. Nutrition and beauty are strongly intertwined, and through a proper diet, you'll be able to show off rejuvenated and radiant skin. If you would like to supplement, it may be useful to know that certain supplements favor skin rejuvenation more than others. Below you'll find the top supplements that will help every woman age gracefully.

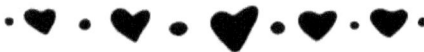

· ♥ · ♥ · ♥ · ♥ · ♥ ·

Vitamin A

You may have heard Vitamin A being described as a supernutrient. This description is quite apt as the vitamin holds many benefits for the immune system and skin. It is present in dairy, spinach, liver, and foods rich in beta-carotene. We will encounter different forms of Vitamin A in many cosmetic products. There are two types of Vitamin A.

- ***Preformed Vitamin A:*** Found in beef, poultry, fish, and dairy. Retinol, retinal and retinoic acid are part of this group.

- ***Provitamin A:*** We find this chiefly in fruits and vegetables. The most common type is beta-carotene.

Regardless if the vitamin is of animal or plant origin, we need enough Vitamin A to remain healthy and support the skin. It is generally recommended that men over 19 years can take a daily dose of 900 micrograms. For women over 19, the recommended daily dose is 700 micrograms. Adolescents are advised to take 600 micrograms, while the dosage in children should not exceed 300 micrograms. It is always recommended to consult a professional when considering Vitamin A. The results depend on correct dosing since taking too little or too much can have counterproductive effects.

Skin Benefits

Vitamin A has some amazing effects on the skin. It encourages healing, smoothes skin, reinforces the skin's natural defenses, and combats free radicals. All of this results in beautiful skin. The anti-aging effects of Vitamin A are well-known, but there are a few other benefits as well.

- *Softer Skin.* Vitamin A promotes skin healing, which pleasantly results in soft skin. It promotes collagen production, making it a great choice to maintain the skin's firmness.

- *Keeps the Skin Hydrated.* Retinoic acid, which is an active form of retinol in our skin, helps to maintain the smoothness of our skin. When our bodies are deficient in this vitamin, dry, itchy skin can be the result.

- *Maintains a Youthful Appearance.* Vitamin A is included in many cosmetic products, which is ascribable to its rejuvenating abilities. Different forms of the vitamin can help to fight wrinkles and spots for an even complexion.

- *The Secret Behind a Perfect Tan.* Beta-carotene can help us develop a more even tan. Don't forget the sunscreen though!

- *Helps to Fight Acne.* Adequate doses of Vitamin A can be very effective in the fight against pimples, blackheads, and comedones. Vitamin A regulates sebum production, leaving the skin smoother (Danti, 2021).

Vitamin A Deficiency

Night blindness is often one of the first signs that you may need more Vitamin A in your life. Severe cases of Vitamin A deficiency can contribute to blindness. In these cases the cornea becomes very dry and damages the retina and cornea (WHO, n.d.). Other signs include dry skin, dry eyes, trouble conceiving, frequent throat and chest infections, poor wound healing, and acne.

Taking too much Vitamin A can be dangerous and is best done under the supervision of a professional.

Selenium

This essential mineral acts on the thyroid system and is involved in fat metabolism. The daily recommended intake of selenium is between 50 and 60 micrograms for adult men and women (Sanchez-Monge, 2019). Selenium can be found in many foods, especially whole grains, fish, seafood, meats, onions, asparagus, Brazil nuts, and sunflower seeds.

Under normal circumstances selenium deficiency will be rare, but it can manifest as heart damage, joint stiffness, swelling, and pain. We need to be careful when supplementing, as too much selenium can lead to changes in the skin, digestive changes, and the loss of teeth.

Selenium benefits the skin by ensuring it remains firm and protected. It stops free radical damage to prevent premature wrinkles from forming and keeps cell membranes safe from UV damage (La Roche-Posay, n.d.). The mineral promotes skin healing and can reduce the appearance of acne.

Vitamin E

Skin care would not be the same without Vitamin E. Its rejuvenating properties are well known. As a powerful antioxidant, Vitamin E protects the skin from free radicals. We get exposed to the cell-damaging agents each day through pollution, cigarette smoke, and UV damage. Vitamin E serves as a bit of a protective shield against these agents.

The Vitamin E used in most cosmetic products is called alpha-tocopherol. Whenever we see "tocopherol" on the ingredients list, we know that Vitamin E is in there. It is recommended that adults consume 15 mg of Vitamin E daily. That is equivalent to one tablespoon of wheat germ oil. Deficiencies are rare and usually related to gastrointestinal issues. If a deficiency does exist symptoms can manifest as loss of balance, muscle weakness, and damage to the retina (WebMD, n.d.).

Skin Benefits

The vitamin is found in many nuts, seeds, oils, and vegetables, making it easy to add to a diet. Vitamin E repairs cell membranes and can soothe eczema and atopic dermatitis. The anti-aging effect is especially noticeable when used in combination with Vitamin C. These two nutrients speed healing, encourage healthy skin cells, and reduce under-eye wrinkles. With all these benefits, it is understandable why Vitamin E is a key ingredient in many beauty products. Skincare that uses Vitamin E to support cell renewal can result in visibly improved skin tone and texture while reducing dark spots (Levey, 2020).

Topical Use

Vitamin E can be used topically and is present in many anti-aging masks and treatments. It is an effective ingredient because it improves the appearance of the skin.

Possible Side Effects from Supplements

It is generally difficult to ingest too much Vitamin E through a balanced diet. Supplementation is generally safe, except when the recommended dosages are exceeded. Too much Vitamin E can increase the risk of bleeding and hemorrhagic stroke and should not be taken by individuals on anticoagulants, simvastatin, niacin, antiplatelets, or who are undergoing radiotherapy or chemotherapy. Always consult your physician first.

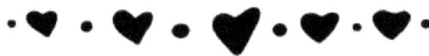

·♥ · ♥ · ♥ · ♥ · ♥ ·

Zinc

It helps the production of new cells and acts in the formation of collagen. Furthermore, zinc repairs damaged tissues and healing wounds. It is also useful to treat irritations and skin injuries. Zinc contributes to maintaining the health of skin, hair, and nails and strengthens the immune system.

A zinc deficiency can contribute to slower wound healing, skin lesions, and white spots on the nails. Restrictive diets and certain health conditions can contribute to zinc deficiency. Too much zinc is also a bad thing. High doses can lead to copper deficiency over time. A weakened immune system and different iron levels are common outcomes as well. Some people may experience low blood pressure or a metallic taste in the mouth, which is why zinc's daily limit of seven milligrams for women and nine milligrams for men should not be exceeded.

There are several foods rich in zinc. Shellfish, nuts, whole grains, meat, fish, legumes, and milk are good sources. Keep in mind that our bodies can only absorb a limited amount of zinc. If it is an agreeable option, try to incorporate zinc of animal origin into your diet. Our bodies use zinc of animal origin a little better than plant origin. Vitamin C and proteins help with zinc absorption.

Ascorbic Acid

Another widely used ingredient in skincare products, ascorbic acid (also called Vitamin C) is used to build blood vessels, collagen, muscle, and cartilage. It is also a vital component in the healing process. This antioxidant helps the body absorb and store iron. Vitamin C is famously found in citrus, berries, tomatoes, peppers, spinach and potatoes. A healthy diet will provide most people with enough Vitamin C. Smokers, selective eaters who avoid fruits and vegetables, and individuals with health issues are more likely to develop a deficiency. Severe Vitamin C deficiency is also called scurvy. It was the bane of the high seas for good reason, causing bleeding gums, poor wound healing, and bruising.

The recommended dosage is 75 milligrams for adult women and 90 milligrams for adult men. Vitamin C usage is generally safe when daily limits are not exceeded. Taking too much can cause nausea, heartburn, headache, stomach cramps, or kidney stones as a result.

Vitamin C supplementation can be harmful to people with kidney problems as it can interact with their medications. The vitamin also interacts with oral contraceptives and certain hormone replacement therapies and may cause estrogen levels to increase as a result (Mayo Clinic, 2018).

Skin Benefits

Ascorbic acid is a skin-loving ingredient that offers many benefits. Commonly used in brightening creams and serums, this vitamin can help to even out skin tone and address dark spots. It is widely used in anti-aging treatments for its ability to reduce expression lines and regenerate the skin.

Vitamin C can help you get the most out of hyaluronic acid serums. Simply use equal amounts of Vitamin C serum and hyaluronic acid serum as you normally would. The results will surprise you.

Some people are sensitive to Vitamin C, but that does not mean that they need to miss out on its benefits. Recently, a new ingredient in skin care products has been drawing more attention due to its powerful antioxidant properties. That ingredient is pycnogenol. This ingredient can be useful to help recycle oxidized Vitamin C products. It can prevent Vitamin C serum from taking an orange tint if a few drops of pycnogenol are mixed in. Pycnogenol can help to reduce pigmentation and boost collagen production, but it is gentler on the skin than Vitamin C.

Pycnogenol is best used in serum form. Use it like you would a Vitamin C serum, once a day in the morning. It can be used in combination with a Vitamin C serum for amped-up protection. Pycnogenol is generally well-tolerated on sensitive skin, but if you have a known pine allergy it is best to steer clear. Try a patch test on the inside of your elbow before using it on your face. Pycnogenol can be found in creams and other skincare products. Skincare products aimed at sensitive skin types may include it among the ingredients.

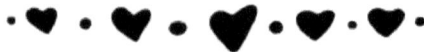

·♥·♥·♥·♥·♥·

Folic Acid

Vitamin B9 (or folic acid) is a water-soluble vitamin. There are many fruits and vegetables rich in this nutrient, which plays a role in cell division. It is best to take folic acid and Vitamin B12 together. These vitamins have a close relationship with the production of red blood cells and iron absorption.

Vitamin B9 encourages cell regeneration and can make the skin more luminous. It reduces small wrinkles and is a powerful anti-aging agent. The vitamin can help to prevent acne and spots and maintain adequate hydration levels in the skin. As a bonus, folic acid makes hair voluminous and strong. Furthermore, it improves firmness by stimulating collagen production and can reduce sun damage.

When we are deficient in folic acid we may experience abundant hair loss and hair thinning. Even though excess folic acid is removed from the body in urine, it is not advisable to overdo it. In rare cases, excess folic acid can trigger skin rashes, digestive problems, gassiness, and other problems. Healthy adults should not exceed a daily dose of 300 micrograms. Folic acid can be taken on its own or as part of a multivitamin.

Vitamin D

Our skin uses sunlight to create Vitamin D. Known for its role in healthy bones and teeth, Vitamin D holds some surprising benefits for your skin. Vitamin D boosts the skin's immune function and reinforces the skin's barrier to prevent moisture loss. Topical applications can help to soothe irritated skin and treat spots. If you find your skin is reacting to topical applications of Vitamin D, it's best to stop usage and consult a professional.

The vitamin is naturally found in fish, egg yolks, and dairy, but supplements are available. A daily dose not exceeding 100 micrograms should be sufficient for most individuals.

Despite being the "Sun Vitamin," it is estimated that 70% of Hispanics are deficient in Vitamin D to some degree (Bjarnadottir, 2021). Vitamin D deficiency can show up as muscle weakness, bone loss, and an increased risk of fractures. Vitamin D deficiency is linked to many health problems.

Too much Vitamin D is associated with symptoms of nausea and weakness. In some cases, kidney stones can develop.

Vitamin K

This vitamin helps the body build healthy bones and tissues and plays a role in blood clotting. This explains why a lack of Vitamin K is associated with heavy bleeding, often starting from the gums or nose. It is a fat-soluble vitamin and there are two types.

- *Vitamin K1:* Plays a role in blood coagulation and is found in leafy green vegetables.

- *Vitamin K2:* Produced in the large intestine, this vitamin helps to create stronger bones and is present in dairy products.

The recommended daily dose for Vitamin K is 90 micrograms for women and 120 micrograms for men.

Vitamin K is used in the treatment of irritated skin and can be useful to remove dark circles (Vanitatis, 2018). It is generally used to resolve problems where an increase in blood supply is involved.

Omega Fatty Acids

Omega fatty acids affect the body on many levels and are present in many foods. These fatty acids help to improve cell structure and lock moisture in the skin. They play a role in repairing the skin's barrier function. This is great news for sensitive skin. These nutrients reduce inflammation and can help the skin feel less sensitive. Omega fatty acids help to repair damage caused by UV rays more quickly and can prevent scaling. These fatty acids are found in oils, nuts, fish, and vegetables.

If you are interested in adding omega fatty acids to your diet through oils, you'll need to keep in mind that humidity, temperature, and light affect the quality of the product. The composition of fatty acids can vary significantly between vegetable oils, and some oils are created artificially.

When we are deficient in omega fatty acids, some interesting signs can arise. A person may experience skin irritation and dryness, mood changes (or feelings of depression), dry eyes, joint pain, and increased shedding and hair loss. Individuals who steer clear of fish and seafood are at an increased risk of deficiency.

There is no recommended daily intake for Omega-6 and 9; however, women can take up to 1.4 grams and men 1.6 grams of Omega-3 daily.

Some side effects of increased omega fatty acid intake may include minor stomach upsets and nausea. If nausea persists, it is best to reduce the dosage. Allergic reactions are rare, but you'll need medical help if itching, swelling, or a rash appears.

Copper

Copper has long enjoyed a reputation for youthfulness in the skincare community. The topical application of copper peptides functions as an antioxidant and can encourage collagen and elastin production. It has anti-inflammatory properties, making it a great option for treating scarring, pigmentation, and redness.

Copper plays a role in our skin and hair color. When we become deficient in copper our skin loses its elasticity, making it easy for dreadful stretch marks to form. The lack of skin elasticity can be caused by a deficiency in Vitamins C, E, B5, and zinc, in addition to copper. Therefore a healthy, balanced diet goes a long way towards retaining the skin's youthfulness. Natural sources of copper include shellfish, shrimp, whole wheat, prunes, beans, and liver.

Common signs that you may need more copper in your life include feeling fatigued or weak, getting sick frequently, having difficulty learning or experiencing memory problems, increased sensitivity to the cold, pale skin, premature gray hair, and in some cases vision loss.

A medical professional will take a health history and may order a blood test to diagnose copper deficiency.

Your risk for copper deficiency increases if you use supplements with zinc in excess, have had bariatric surgery, or suffer from certain health conditions.

Supplementing with copper can be harmful if you take too much. Too much copper can lead to liver damage, nausea, cramps, and abdominal pain. Therefore it is recommended to stay within the daily limits of 15 mg for men and 12 mg for women (Bailey, n.d.).

Coenzyme Q10

More than a trendy ingredient in anti-aging products, Q10 is a natural ally in our fight to delay the signs of aging. Coenzyme Q10 occurs naturally in the body and contributes to the functioning of cells. One of its main functions is to energize cells, facilitating cell regeneration. It also acts as a powerful antioxidant to preserve the youthful radiance of our skin for much longer.

Food sources of Q10 can be found in poultry, sardines, eggs, potatoes, leafy greens, and legumes. A daily dose of 90 to 200 mg of the coenzyme is typically recommended (Kubala, 2018) if supplementing. Your skin care regimen can enhance the effects. Make sure to use skincare products with Q10 as an ingredient. The results will surprise you.

Q10 delays aging, which makes it a much-loved ingredient in beauty products. By energizing cells and stimulating cell regeneration, the natural structure of the skin becomes reinforced, visibly reducing wrinkles. Q10 also helps the skin maintain firmness and smoothness.

Another benefit that is not talked about enough is Q10's ability to make other nutrients work harder. When Q10 is used in combination with Vitamin C and E, their antioxidant and collagen production effects are enhanced (de Sevilla, 2021). The results are beautifully radiant skin.

Mild cases of coenzyme Q10 deficiency can cause problems with coordination in our late 60s (MedLine Plus, n.d.-c). Take Q10 in smaller doses instead of one big dose. Smaller doses throughout the day can help to reduce the side effects. The average daily dose ranges from 100 to 200 milligrams. It is best to get advice from a professional.

Sulfur

This trace element helps out with metabolism. It is present in protein-rich foods and a balanced diet provides all you need (Martinez Blasco, 2015). Sulfur has many cosmetic uses and can improve skin elasticity. It eliminates accumulated toxins in the skin and can soothe allergies. Sulfur also evens out skin pigmentation.

Sulfur is used to treat many skin conditions and is present in bars, lotions, and creams to treat acne. Those suffering from allergies may benefit from adding sulfur-rich foods to their diet. Natural sources include mango, fish, shellfish, and onion to name a few. Make sure to use sulfur-containing products only as directed.

When using sulfur containing products, take care to keep them away from your eyes. If you accidentally get some product in your eye, rinse thoroughly. When using sulfur in cream or lotion form, always wash affected areas before application.

Potassium

Our bodies need potassium to stay healthy. Most women need 2,600 milligrams of potassium per day. Men need 3,400 milligrams daily. Add more potassium-rich foods to the diet to prevent deficiencies. Potatoes, bananas, and mushrooms are rich in potassium.

High levels of potassium can be harmful, especially in the elderly and those with kidney problems (American Heart Association, 2018). So be careful with supplements and speak to a professional first. Some salt substitutes can increase the amount of potassium in your diet. These typically contain a lot of potassium and very little sodium.

If your skin feels constantly dry and itchy, despite moisturizing, it may be a sign that your diet is lacking potassium. The mineral regulates water storage in the body and keeps the skin glowing

Potassium supports fast cell renewal, lending a younger and healthier appearance to the skin. The nutrient helps to improve scars and blemishes and maintains the pH balance of the skin. When we have really dry skin, the pH balance may be disrupted. Since potassium helps the skin to retain moisture, the skin remains healthy and balanced for a longer time.

Potassium deficiency may be behind that nagging hair loss. When potassium is in short supply the scalp can dry out, contributing to hair loss. On the flip side, we may experience enhanced hair growth when our diets are rich in potassium.

Silicon

Silicon is an essential ingredient for younger and more elastic skin. This mineral helps to maintain healthy skin and keeps signs of aging at bay. This trace element is naturally present in our bodies and plays a role in collagen and elastin production (Danti, 2017).

The reserves of organic silicon deplete with age, making it necessary to up one's intake of this mineral from age 40. Doing so will help to maintain healthy skin, but the mineral has other benefits too.

- It stimulates collagen protection.

- Has a detoxifying action.

- Strengthens cartilage.

- Improves skin problems and sunburn.

- Protects the skin against free radicals and wrinkles.

Silicon can be found in whole grains and several other vegetables and is a staple in beauty products.

Magnesium

The times when our skin looks dull or damaged may point to a magnesium deficiency. Many people consume less than the recommended daily amount (RDA). The RDA for an adult woman is 310 mg. Whole grains, leafy greens, and legumes are excellent dietary sources.

Magnesium makes the skin look stunning. It helps to maintain a healthy skin barrier and can be used topically. It is often included in anti-inflammatory products and cosmetics. Up to 40% of dietary magnesium is absorbed by the body (Women's Health, 2016). If you are supplementing, it can be easy to overdo it. Side effects from too much magnesium may include diarrhea. In extreme cases, too much magnesium can be deadly.

To avoid an overdose, it is best to look for a multivitamin that contains magnesium, Vitamin D3, calcium, and iron. These vitamins will balance each other out. Slow-release vitamins are a good option.

Niacinamides

Better known as Vitamin B3, this essential water-soluble nutrient ensures that our cells stay healthy. Our bodies can't produce it, so it becomes necessary to include eggs, legumes, fish, and other food sources in our diets.

The most dramatic effects of niacinamide can be seen in topical applications. The vitamin is used in cosmetics and is easily absorbed by the skin. Vitamin B3 is believed to be useful in treating acne and eczema. It protects the skin barrier and has soothing and firming properties. The antioxidant properties cannot be overlooked either. The vitamin can help reduce the signs of aging, lighten dark spots to even skin tone and encourage collagen production.

If you are supplementing, it is recommended to limit your intake to 35 grams per day for adults.

Thiamine

Better known as Vitamin B1, this nutrient has benefits for acne-prone and dry skin. It also can improve the appearance of wrinkles. It does this by aiding cell reproduction, enabling us to have clear and healthy skin.

Thiamine is often included in products aimed at managing acne. When taken orally, adult men should not exceed a daily dose of 1.2 mg. Adult women are advised to take 1 mg daily.

If you suffer from stress-related breakouts, thiamine may be able to help. The vitamin is known as the "anti-stress" vitamin and can calm the nervous system. Simply include thiamine-rich foods like sunflower seeds, legumes, seeds, and mussels in your diet. If you go the supplement route, don't exceed the daily recommended dose.

Riboflavin

Another member of the B-vitamin family, riboflavin is also called Vitamin B2. This vitamin is important for cells to grow and develop and plays a role in converting food to energy. The amount of Vitamin B2 you will need will depend on your age and gender. Generally, adult women will need 1.1 micrograms daily (National Institutes of Health, n.d.).

The vitamin is found in many foods including eggs, lean meat, and certain vegetables. If the supplement route is more your speed, riboflavin is typically found in multivitamin and Vitamin B-complex dietary products. Deficiency in Vitamin B2 is quite uncommon, but strict vegans, pregnant women, and those who don't consume dairy products are more likely to develop a deficiency.

When there is a shortage of riboflavin, we may develop tears in the corner of the mouth, painful cracked lips, and hair loss. Sometimes anemia can settle in if the deficiency is significant enough.

Pantothenic Acid

Vitamin B5 is water-soluble and plays a role in the production of antibodies. Vitamin B5 helps keep the skin moisturized and can reduce acne-related blemishes. When we are deficient in this vitamin, symptoms may present as insomnia, fatigue, stress, migraines, or even numbness in the hands and feet. A balanced diet provides us with all the Vitamin B5 we need. Rich dietary sources include brewer's yeast, cauliflower, avocado, salmon, and cheese. The skin draws several benefits from this vitamin.

- *Keeps Moisture in the Skin:* Vitamin B5 helps to control water loss from the skin. Problems like dry skin, itchiness, and flakiness can be improved.

- ***Works as an Anti-inflammatory:*** When applied topical-ly, it can help to protect the skin from redness caused by sun exposure.

- ***Makes Scars Less Visible:*** Topical application (a serum, cream, or gel) can reduce scar visibility.

- ***Is an Antioxidant:*** B5 is a powerful antioxidant and fights the signs of aging on a deeper level in the skin. Vitamin B5 targets wrinkles where they form, in the middle layer of the skin, to boost collagen and elastin production.

The recommended daily dose is six milligrams for healthy adults (Nutritienda, 2009). The vitamin is considered to be safe, but large doses may cause diarrhea.

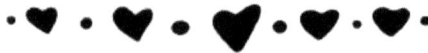

•♥ • ♥ • ♥ • ♥ • ♥ •

Biotin

Eggs, liver, and avocado are rich sources of Vitamin B7. The nutrient helps our enzymes function properly and plays a role in regenerating our skin and hair (Navarro, 2021b). This makes biotin a popular ingredient in skincare products.

The vitamin encourages blood circulation and helps to regulate oil production. People with oily and combination skin are encouraged to add biotin-rich foods to their diet. The vitamin helps to regulate oil production. As a bonus, it makes the hair more voluminous. The recommended daily dose for adult men and women is 30 micrograms.

Biotin is water-soluble, so it does not lead to toxicity, but there is a side effect to be mindful of. Large quantities can lead to a decrease of Vitamin B5. Sticking within the recommended daily allowance usually averts this problem.

Vitamin F

The name is a bit of a misnomer. Vitamin F is not a vitamin, it is a mixture of fatty acids. In skin care products, it acts as a moisturizer and prevents aging. It prevents scaling and assists in skin repair. Skin-care products, milks, and shampoo formulated for dry hair tend to include Vitamin F as an ingredient, and for good reason. It improves hydration, reduces redness, and gives the skin a luminous glow. Acne, aging, and blemish treatments make use of the vitamin's oil-controlling abilities. A balanced diet rich in Omega-3 generally provides all the fatty acids you'd need.

Iron

Dark circles under the eyes and pale skin are common signs of anemia. It is caused by iron deficiency. Iron is needed to transport oxygen throughout the body. It is also essential in making connective tissues and hormones, making it a necessary nutrient for glowing skin.

There are two types of dietary sources. Heme iron and non-heme iron, i.e. iron of animal origin or plant origin. Animal origin iron is better absorbed by the body. If your main iron source is mostly plant-based, it is advisable to take Vitamin C to improve absorption. The typical recommendation for an adult woman is 18 mg. Individual needs may vary, so it is a good idea to speak to a professional before turning to supplements.

When your iron intake is too high you may experience gastric discomfort or constipation. Excessively high iron intake is linked to organ failure and can damage the liver.

Polyphenols

Found in plants, these powerful antioxidants protect the skin against sun damage. They are used as natural preservatives in cosmetics and have powerful anti-aging effects. Polyphenols help the skin maintain its firmness. When applied topically, they can repair and rejuvenate the skin. They can prevent some forms of sun damage and reverse many signs of aging. Use a polyphenol-packed serum and broad-spectrum sunscreen every morning. The polyphenols will boost your sunscreen's protective powers for better sun protection. Nearly all of our skincare and cosmetic products contain some form of polyphenol.

· ♥ · ♥ · ♥ · ♥ · ♥ ·

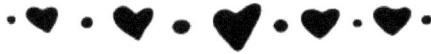

Probiotics and Your Skin

If your skin is acne-prone, probiotics might become a new best friend. They help your skin achieve balance. Probiotics are easily found in yogurt and sauerkraut and have benefits for our digestive health. Our skin may enjoy these benefits:

- *Skin Conditions Improve.* Acne, rashes, and other skin conditions may result when our gut flora is altered. Probiotics help to restore balance, improving the skin conditions that were triggered.

- *Smoother Appearance.* The topical use of probiotics may help to build collagen, which smoothes out the appearance.

- *Better Skin Hydration*. Certain strains of probiotics may help to strengthen the skin barrier. A strong skin barrier is necessary to prevent dryness.

- *Fewer Breakouts.* Probiotics are anti-inflammatory. Regular use, therefore, keeps inflammation at bay, resulting in fewer breakouts.

It is believed that the effects of probiotics are their most potent when ingested. Our health is tied to our gut health and our skin reflects our overall health. Probiotics may help to improve atopic dermatitis by maintaining the natural balance in the gut.

To make the most out of probiotics, we need to include prebiotics. We can think of prebiotics as the "food" for live probiotics. Probiotics ensure that the skin barrier is happy by regulating oil production. Probiotics can combat the damage caused by free radicals, thereby delaying the signs of aging.

The ability of probiotics to rebuild the skin barrier should be of special importance to people with sensitive skin. Sensitive skin takes a bit longer to repair when damaged, but probiotics can help speed up the healing process. Your skin will be less inflamed and irritated as a result.

The topical application of probiotics helps to shield the skin and can be effective in the treatment of acne (Acosta, 2021). Certain skin types favor certain probiotics. Blemish-prone skin can turn to skin care products containing eutropha nitrosomes. Dry skin finds benefits from lactobacillus rhamnosus. Lactobacillus paracasei is beneficial for sensitive skin, while aging and sun-damaged skin can use non-living bifida glycoprotein with good results.

• ♥ • ♥ • ♥ • ♥ • ♥ •

Collagen to Rejuvenate Skin

Collagen is a family of proteins that can be found in connective tissues, organs, skin, and bones. You may spot "hydrolyzed collagen" on the supplement label and wonder what it means. Hydrolyzed collagen is collagen that is broken down into easy-to-process particles. From there, the collagen is broken down into amino acids and used by the body. Collagen supplements can be expensive, but gelatin may prove to be a budget-friendly alternative (Cenizo, 2017).

Collagen can account for nearly seven percent of a person's body mass, and plays a leading role in our skin's fitness and elasticity. Collagen is one of the main components found in the dermis and gives the skin its texture. We can't overlook elastin, though. Elastin gives the skin a youthful appearance and helps to maintain skin hydration. Elastin also plays a role in preventing breaks in connective tissue fibers, dermis, and the epidermis, slowing facial aging.

Skin with healthy levels of collagen and elastin is stronger and more resistant to damage. There are several different types of collagen, which is why the nutrient is sometimes referred to as a "family of proteins." Elastin provides connective tissues the ability to stretch and return to their original shape, lending elasticity to our skin.

- Adequate collagen intake has additional benefits for the skin, granting it a luminous appearance free from signs of fatigue.

- It assists in skin rejuvenation, leaving the skin soft to the touch.

- Collagen is useful in the battle against dry skin. The protein helps to preserve optimal water levels in the skin, keeping it hydrated.

- Collagen famously stops skin sagging and minimizes expression lines. From 35 years of age onwards, our bodies don't produce as much collagen, which may result in early signs of aging. By replenishing our collagen levels, we can make sure the skin retains its youthful appearance for longer.

The protein grants our skin, hair, and nails a healthy appearance and can prevent stretch marks. It plays a big role in the healing process, so introducing collagen-rich foods into your diet may benefit your skin in many ways.

Certain foods are high in collagen, while others contribute to its manufacture in the body. Red fruits and vegetables (tomatoes, strawberries) are useful to stimulate collagen production. Nuts, bone broth, dairy, and foods containing sulfur are good dietary sources of collagen.

There is insufficient evidence to support the use of collagen supplements. As with most nutrients, the best way to benefit from them is through a balanced diet. Supplements are generally safe and the amount of collagen will vary depending on the form. A daily dose of 2.5 grams of hydrolyzed collagen may benefit skin health and hydration. Larger doses are typically used to improve bone density and muscle mass. When using undenatured collagen, a dose of up to 40 mg daily may grant skin and joint benefits. Undenatured collagen differs from hydrolyzed collagen slightly. Here the collagen is still in a biologically active form, whereas in the hydrolyzed form it is broken down into peptides. It is possible to boost collagen intake without supplements, but the data is limited on gelatin's efficacy when used as a supplement. The form of cooked collagen is frequently added to sauces, soups, and gelatinous desserts, but there are no specific dosage recommendations available.

It's important to remember that UV light breaks down collagen. Wearing sunscreen and enjoying a diet rich in antioxidants are two of the best ways you can preserve your collagen levels naturally.

There is a bit of debate about whether biotin or collagen is better for your skin. When we are biotin deficient, supplementing with the vitamin can help to improve skin health. But, in general, collagen seems to be the better option for improving the skin's appearance.

When a person has a biotin deficiency, taking a supplement may improve the health of their skin. Otherwise, collagen can be a better option as there is more evidence to suggest it helps improve the skin's appearance. Studies investigating how collagen delays the aging process have found encouraging results, pointing towards collagen as the supplement of choice to delay aging. Biotin, on the other hand, has no studies to back it up yet. Still, it is perfectly safe to take biotin and collagen together.

· ❤ · ❤ · ❤ · ❤ · ❤ ·

Conclusion

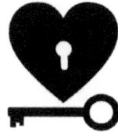

ood skin care is a daily habit that grows and changes along
with your skin's specific needs. Now you know that the skin
requires different steps to treat it, according to its type, age, color, and
even internal and external factors, so a standard solution has never
worked. This book aims to give you the tools to know your skin and
solve all possible threats that may cause imperfections on your face.

We all deserve to have healthy skin. However, imperfections show us
that something is amiss. We must act in time to correct blemishes
and skin challenges with knowledge. After all, who better than you
to identify what your skin needs?

At present, the multiple talents that Latina women have made us
successful protagonists on several fronts. Interaction at a social and
professional level has become indispensable and present in our lives,
especially in recent decades. This book is for us who have empowered
ourselves daily in values, knowledge, and image. As part of this set,
having beautiful skin becomes an asset and a fantastic confidence
boost. It is also an excellent reason to take better care of our bodies.
The condition of our skin is tied to nutrition, our commitment to
wearing sunscreen, and providing proper daily care.

You now understand that effective skin care depends on one or more specific goals. For example, some people want to age gracefully, while others want to address sensitivity and control excess oil production.

This book serves as a guide to women like you or me. Learning to care for your skin is a journey as you mature. As a result, the actions you apply today may be different for you in the future, and you may need to refresh your memory of the lessons learned.

Remember that the best gifts are those that last in our minds and are part of our daily routine.

A big hug!

Artemixbeauty

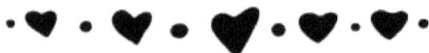

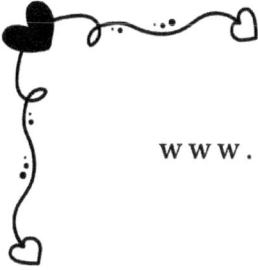

www.artemixbeauty.com

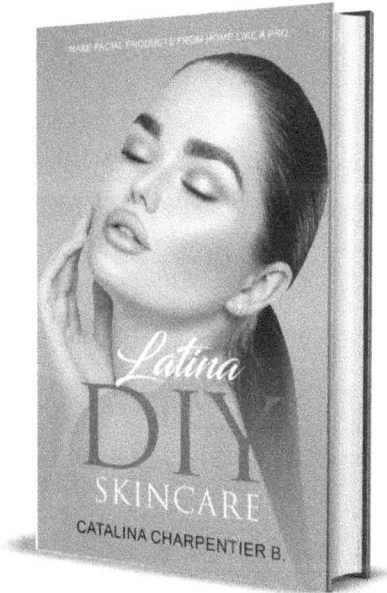

Take your Skincare to the next level! Discover how to create natural products like a professional from the comfort of your home.

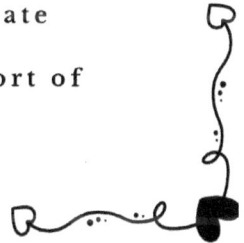

I feel proud to write for our Latino community.

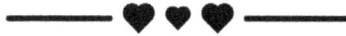

———— ♥ ♥ ♥ ————

If you enjoyed reading my book, please leave me your review and recommend it. Your opinion is precious to me, as it motivates me to continue researching and developing knowledge that meets our specific needs.

Hughs.
Catalina

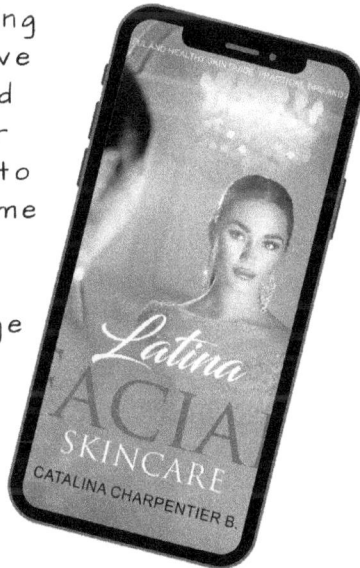

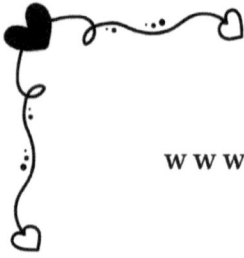

www.artemixbeauty.com

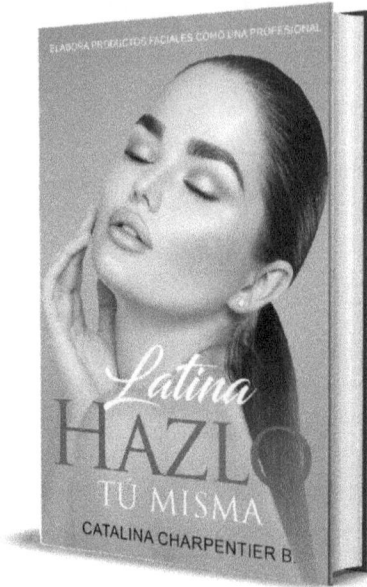

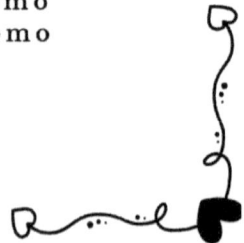

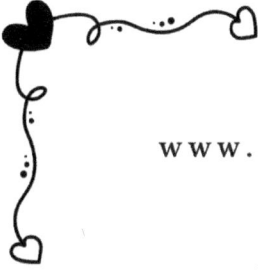

www.artemixbeauty.com

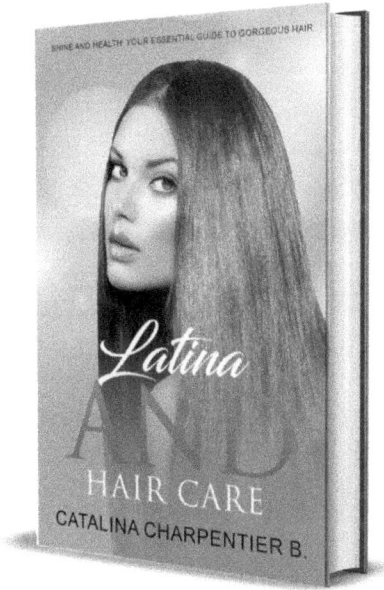

Descubre los secretos para lucir espectacular en cada página. Aprende sobre el cuidado de la piel, la elección de productos y los mejores suplementos para rejuvenecer tu rostro.

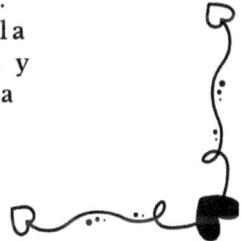

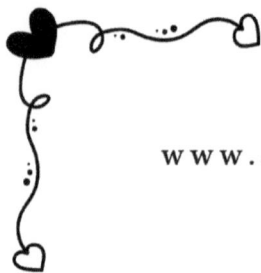

www.artemixbeauty.com

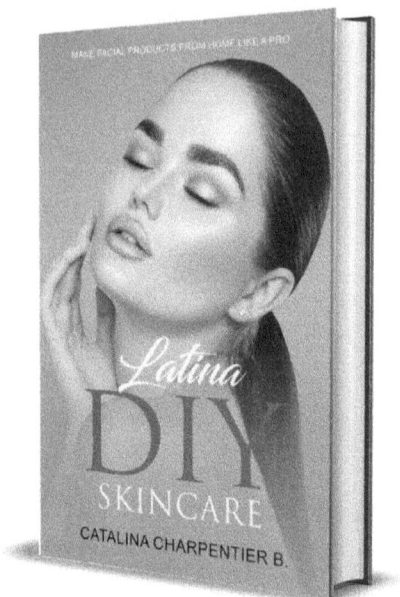

Take your Skincare to the next level! Discover how to create natural products like a professional from the comfort of your home.

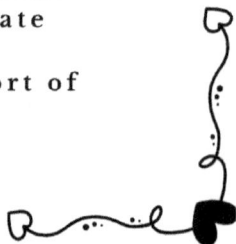

References

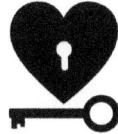

Acosta, L. (2021, July 7). *¿Sabías que los probióticos pueden transformar tu piel?* People En Español. https://peopleenespanol.com/pon te-bella/probioticos-prebioticos-postbioticos-transforma-tu-piel/

American Cancer Society. (n.d.). *Cancer facts & figures for Hispanics/Latinos 2012-2014.* Retrieved June 4, 2022, https://www.cancer.org/content/dam/cancer-org/research/cancer-f acts-and-statistics/cancer-facts-and-figures-for-hispanics-and-latinos /cancer-facts-and-figures-for-hispanics-and-latinos-2012-2014.pdf

American Cancer Society. (2019). *Factores de riesgo para el cáncer de piel tipo melanoma.* American Cancer Society. https://www.cancer.org/es/cancer/cancer-de-piel-tipo-melano ma/causas-riesgos-prevencion/factores-de-riesgo.html

American Cancer Society. (2022, January 12). *Estadísticas importantes sobre el cáncer de piel tipo melanoma.* American Cancer Society. https://www.cancer.org/es/cancer/cancer-de-piel-tipo-melan oma/acerca/estadisticas-clave.html

American Heart Association. (2018, May 24). *A primer on potassium*. Www.goredforwomen.org. https://www.goredforwomen.org/es/healthy-living/healthy-eating/eat-smart/sodium/potassium

Andrades, P., Benítez, S., & Prado, A. (2006). Recomendaciones para el manejo de cicatrices hipertróficas y queloides. *Revista Chilena de Cirugía, 58*(2), 78–88. https://doi.org/10.4067/S0718-402620060 00200003

Bailey, J. (n.d.). *How to take copper with zinc*. LIVESTRONG.COM. Retrieved June 17, 2022, from https://www.livestrong.com/article /511087-how-to-take-copper-with-zinc/

Bard, S. (2021, September 21). *Eczema and stress: Triggers, connection, and more*. Www.medicalnewstoday.com . https://www.medicalnewstoday.com/articles/eczema-and-stress#: ~:text=A%202020%20prospective%20study%20looked

Begoun, P. (n.d.). *Face scrubs: Everything you need to know*. Paula's Choice Skincare. https://www.paulaschoice.com/expert-advice/ski ncare-advice/cleansers/to-scrub-or-not-to-scrub.html

Benedetti, J. (2022, January). *Photosensitivity reactions - Skin disorders*. MSD Manual Consumer Version. https://www.msdmanuals.com/home/skin-disorders/sunlight-and -skin-damage/photosensitivity-reactions#:~:text=Photosensitivity% 2C%20sometimes%20referred%20to%20as

Bjarnadottir, A. (2021, February 15). *How much Vitamin D should you take for optimal health?* Healthline. https://www.healthline.com/nutrition/how-much-vitamin-d -to-take#How-common-is-vitamin-D-deficiency?

Borve, A. (2017, April 8). *La Academia Americana de Dermatología evalúa el riesgo de cáncer de piel en latinos.* First Derm. https://www.firstderm.com/es/la-acael-riesgo-de-cancer-de-piel-en-latinos/

Brooks, C. J., Gortmaker, S. L., Long, M. W., Cradock, A. L., & Kenney, E. L. (2017). Racial/Ethnic and Socioeconomic Disparities in Hydration Status Among US Adults and the Role of Tap Water and Other Beverage Intake. *American Journal of Public Health, 107*(9), 1387–1394. https://doi.org/10.2105/ajph.2017.303923

Cantu-Pawlik, S. (2019, June 14). *Latino kids face chronic skin condition disparities.* Salud America. https://salud-america.org/latinos-face-chronic-skin-condition-disparities-eczema/#:~:text=Latinos%20are%20among%20those%20groups

Carswell, L., & Borger, J. (2020). *Hypertrophic scarring keloids.* PubMed; StatPearls Publishing. https://www.ncbi.nlm.nih.gov/books/NBK537058/

Cenizo, N. (2017, October 5). *Colágeno para deportistas: ¿Sirve para algo el suplemento de moda?* Salud Más Deporte. Expertos En Medicina Deportiva Y Deporte Saludable. https://www.saludmasdeporte.com/colageno-hidrolizado-articulaciones/

Cobb, C. (2022, April 25). *Dark circles under your eyes: Causes and treatments.* Healthline. https://www.healthline.com/health/dark-circle-under-eyes#causes

Cronan, K. (n.d.). *Cómo escoger y usar un protector solar (para Padres) - Nemours KidsHealth*. Nemours Children's Health. https://kidsh ealth.org/es/parents/sunscreen.html

CuídatePlus Editorial Office. (2017, October 18). *¿Sabes reconocer tu tipo de piel?* CuidatePlus. https://cuidateplus.marca.com/belleza-y-piel/cuidados-f aciales/2017/10/20/-reconocer-tipo-piel-145874.html

Danti, C. M. (2017, August 16). *Propiedades del silicio para la piel - ideal para eliminar la flacidez.* Www.mundodeportivo.com/Uncomo. https://www.mundodeportivo.com/uncomo/belleza/articulo/pro piedades-del-silicio-para-la-piel-ideal-para-eliminar-la-flacidez-4686 5.html#:~:text=Silicio%20en%20cosm%C3%A9tica

Danti, C. M. (2021, March 19). *Vitamina A para la piel: beneficios, alimentos y cómo tomarla.* Www.mundodeportivo.com/Uncomo. https://www.mundodeportivo.com/uncomo/belleza/articulo/vita mina-a-para-la-piel-beneficios-alimentos-y-como-tomarla-51112.ht ml

de Sevilla, D. (2021, October 2). *Qué es la coenzima Q10 y por qué es la mejor aliada contra el envejecimiento.* Diario de Sevilla. https://www.diariodesevilla.es/wappissima/belleza/que-es-coen zima-Q10-contra-envejecimiento_0_1615638895.html

Duke University. (2019, June 26). *What made humans "the fat primate"? Changes in DNA packaging curbed our body's ability to turn "bad" fat into "good" fat.* ScienceDaily. https://www.sciencedaily.c om/releases/2019/06/190626160337.htm

Eucerin. (n.d.-a). *Atopic dermatitis on the face - causes & treatment | Eucerin*. Www.eucerin.co.za. Retrieved June 16, 2022, from https://www.eucerin.co.za/skin-concerns/atopic-dermatitis/facial-a topic-dermatitis#:~:text=The%20symptoms%20of%20facial%20At opic

Eucerin. (n.d.-b). *Eucerin: Hypersensitive, redness-prone skin | Hypersensitivity in general*. Eucerin. Retrieved June 6, 2022, from https://int.eucerin.com/skin-concerns/hypersensitive-redness-pron e-skin/hypersensitivity-in-general#:~:text=Hypersensitive%20skin% 20%2D%20or%20very%20sensitive

Eucerin. (n.d.-c). *Eucerin: Piel atópica | Dermatitis atópica facial*. Www.eucerin.es. Retrieved June 15, 2022, from https://www.eucerin.es/problemas-de-la-piel/dermatitis-atopica/de rmatitis-atopica-en-la-cara#:~:text=La%20dermatitis%20at%C3%B 3pica%20(o%20eccema

Evans, S. (2022, May 20). *How to use a face mask the right way - L'Oréal Paris*. L'Oréal Paris. https://www.lorealparisusa.com/beauty-magazine/skin-care/ skin-care-essentials/face-mask-mistakes-to-avoid

Farmacia Maiz Piat. (2019, November 30). *Cómo prevenir y tratar las manchas de la cara*. Www.farmaciamaizpiat.es. https://www.farma ciamaizpiat.es/blog/como-prevenir-y-tratar-las-manchas-de-la-cara

FDA. (2018, November 3). *Sun Protection Factor (SPF)*. FDA. https://www.fda.gov/about-fda/center-drug-evaluation-and -research-cder/sun-protection-factor-spf

Gauglitz, G. G., Korting, H. C., Pavicic, T., Ruzicka, T., & Jeschke, M. G. (2011). Hypertrophic scarring and keloids: pathomechanisms and current and emerging treatment strategies. *Molecular Medicine (Cambridge, Mass.)*, *17*(1-2), 113–125. https://doi.org/10.2119/m olmed.2009.00153

Gil, P. A. (2022, March 27). *Acné adulto: qué es y cómo combatir la aparición de granos*. Esquire. https://www.esquire.com/es/cuidado s-hombre/a39492062/acne-adulto-hombre-tratamiento/

Goulden, V., Clark, S. M., & Cunliffe, W. J. (1997). Post-adolescent acne: a review of clinical features. *The British Journal of Dermatology*, *136*(1), 66–70. https://pubmed.ncbi.nlm.nih.gov/9039297/

Guarino, D. F. (2021, March 4). *Acné en la mujer adulta: causas, características y tratamiento*. Madriderma. https://madriderma.co m/acne-mujer-adulta/

Hand, J. (2017, March 22). *Opciones de tratamiento para las cicatrices del acné que no mejoran con el tiempo*. Red de Noticias de Mayo   Clinic. https://newsnetwork.mayoclinic.org/es/2017/03/22/opciones-de-t ratamiento-para-las-cicatrices-del-acne-que-no-mejoran-con-el-tiem po/

Henríquez, M. P., Karla. (2018, March 16). *Entiende el fun-cionamiento de las cremas antiarrugas*. Mejor Con Salud. https://m ejorconsalud.as.com/entiende-funcionamiento-cremas-antiarrugas/

Jablonski, N. G. (1999). A possible link between neural tube defects and ultraviolet light exposure. *Medical Hypotheses, 52*(6), 581–582. https://doi.org/10.1054/mehy.1997.0697

Jablonski, N. G., & Chaplin, G. (2013). Epidermal pigmentation in the human lineage is an adaptation to ultraviolet radiation. *Journal of Human Evolution, 65*(5), 671–675. https://doi.org/10.1016/j.jhevol.2013.06.004

Kaufman, B., & Alexis, A. (2018, February 16). *Eczema in skin of color: What you need to know.* National Eczema Association. https://nationaleczema.org/blog/eczema-in-skin-of-color/

Kirchweger, G. (2001). The Biology of Skin Color: Black and White. *Discover, 22*(2).

Kowalczyk, J. (2020, May). *How atopic dermatitis can harm your mental health.* Sharecare. https://www.sharecare.com/skin-health/atopic-dermatitis-mental-health?cbr=ggle11202021

Kubala, J. (2018, September 4). *CoQ10 Dosage: How much should you take per day?* Healthline; Healthline Media. https://www.healthline.com/nutrition/coq10-dosage#dosages

La Roche-Posay. (n.d.). *10 zinc and selenium-rich foods you should eat more often for glowing skin | La Roche Posay UK.* LaRoche-Posay. Retrieved June 16, 2022, from https://www.laroche-posay.co.uk/en_GB/10-zinc-and-selenium-rich-foods-you-should-eat-more-often-for-glowing-skin.html#:~:text=Selenium%20is%20also%20a%20mineral

Levey, D. K. (2020, October 15). *¿Cuáles son los benefi-cios de la vitamina E para mi piel? | La barra*. Neutroge-na. https://es.neutrogena.com/the-bar/the-benefits-of-vitamin-e.h
tml#:~:text=El%20cuidado%20de%20la%20piel

Link, R. (2020, January 28). *5 benefits and uses of micellar wa-ter*. Healthline. https://www.healthline.com/nutrition/micellar-wa
ter-benefits#_noHeaderPrefixedContent

Loomis, W. F. (1967). Skin-Pigment Regulation of Vitamin-D Biosynthesis in Man: Variation in solar ultraviolet at different latitudes may have caused racial differentiation in man. *Science*, *157*(3788), 501–506. https://doi.org/10.1126/science.157.3788.5
01

L'Oreal Paris. (n.d.). *How to cover up acne with makeup*. L'Oréal Paris. Retrieved June 15, 2022, from https://www.lorealparisusa.com/be
auty-magazine/makeup/face-makeup/how-to-cover-up-acne

Lyons, A. B., Moy, L., Moy, R., & Tung, R. (2019). Cir-cadian Rhythm and the Skin: A Review of the Litera-ture. *The Journal of Clinical and Aesthetic Dermatology*, *12*(9), 42–45. https://www.ncbi.nlm.nih.gov/pmc/articles/PMC677769
9/#:~:text=The%20skin%20contains%20circadian%20clock

Martinez Blasco, E. (2015, May 17). *Azufre: usos y beneficios para la salud*. Mejor Con Salud. https://mejorconsalud.as.com/azufre-uso
s-beneficios-la-salud/

Mayo Clinic. (n.d.-a). *Acné - Diagnóstico y tratamiento - Mayo Clinic.* Www.mayoclinic.org. https://www.mayoclinic.org/es-es/diseases-c onditions/acne/diagnosis-treatment/drc-20368048

Mayo Clinic. (n.d.-b). *Dermatitis - Diagnosis and treatment - Mayo Clinic.* Www.mayoclinic.org. https://www.mayoclinic.org/diseases -conditions/dermatitis-eczema/diagnosis-treatment/drc-20352386

Mayo Clinic. (2018). *Vitamina C.* Mayo Clinic. https://www.may oclinic.org/es-es/drugs-supplements-vitamin-c/art-20363932

Mayo Clinic. (2019). *Wrinkle creams: Your guide to younger looking skin.* Mayo Clinic. https://www.mayoclinic.org/diseases-condition s/wrinkles/in-depth/wrinkle-creams/art-20047463

McGill, M. (2018, June 18). *Sun protection factor (SPF): What is the best sunscreen?* Medical News Today. https://www.medicalnewstod ay.com/articles/306838#_noHeaderPrefixedContent

MedLine Plus. (n.d.-a). *Acne - self-care: MedlinePlus Medical Ency-clopedia.* MedLine Plus. https://medlineplus.gov/ency/patientinstr uctions/000750.htm

MedLine Plus. (n.d.-b). *Aging changes in skin: MedlinePlus Medical Encyclopedia.* Medlineplus.gov . https://medlineplus.gov/ency/article/004014.htm#:~:text=With %20aging%2C%20the%20outer%20skin

MedLine Plus. (n.d.-c). *Primary coenzyme Q10 deficiency: MedlinePlus Genetics.* Medlineplus.gov. Retrieved June 17, 2022, f r o m https://medlineplus.gov/genetics/condition/primary-coenzyme-q1

0-deficiency/#:~:text=Primary%20coenzyme%20Q10%20deficiency
%20is

Mukherjee, T. (2019, May 23). *What is skin PH? How to tell if yours is healthy, and why it matters.* EverydayHealth.com. https://www.everydayhealth.com/skin-beauty/skin-ph-yours-health
y-why-it-matters-how-tell/#:~:text=%E2%80%9CThe%20pH%20o
f%20your%20cleansers

Nast, C. (2021a, March 9). *Todo sobre los sérum: para qué sirven, cómo se usan y cuál elegir según tus necesidades.* Vogue España. https://www.vogue.es/belleza/articulos/mejor-serum-com
o-usar-acido-hialuronico-vitamina-c-retinol

Nast, C. (2021b, May 20). *A cada tipo de piel, su limpiador facial perfecto.* Vogue España. https://www.vogue.es/belleza/articulos/limpieza-facial-tipos
-limpiadores-desmaquillantes-cual-elegir-piel-grasa-seca-sensible

Nast, C. (2021c, July 26). *Tónicos faciales: todo lo que necesitas saber de ellos.* Glamour. https://www.glamour.mx/belleza/articulos/ton
icos-faciales-todo-lo-que-necesitas-saber/20994

National Institutes of Health. (n.d.). *Office of Dietary Supplements - Riboflavina.* Ods.od.nih.gov. https://ods.od.nih.gov/factsheets/Riboflavin-DatosEnEspanol/#:~:
text=La%20riboflavina%2C%20conocida%20tambi%C3%A9n%20
como

Navarro, R. M. (2021a, February 18). *¿Qué es una crema despigmentante facial y como debo usarla? • Farmacia Angulo.*

Farmacia   Angulo.
https://nutricionyfarmacia.es/blog/belleza/cara/que-es-una-crema
-despigmentante-como-debo-usarla/#:~:text=Las%20manchas%20e
n%20el%20rostro

Navarro, R. M. (2021b, October 27). *Biotina para el Pelo: Para qué
sirve y Beneficios • Farmacia Angulo.* Farmacia Angulo. https://nut
ricionyfarmacia.es/blog/belleza/pelo/biotina-para-el-pelo/

Nicolas, A. (2019, June 27). *¿Qué es una crema despigmentante y qué
puede hacer por tu piel?* TELVA. https://www.telva.com/belleza/20
19/06/27/5d12a02701a2f14c9b8b4667.html

NORD (National Organization for Rare Disorders). (
n.d.). *Prurigo Nodularis.* NORD (National Organization for Rare Disorders). Retrieved June 16, 2022,
from https://rarediseases.org/rare-diseases/prurigo-nodularis/#:~:t
ext=Prurigo%20nodularis%20(PN)%20is%20a

Nutritienda. (2009, December 31). *¿Pará que sirve el Ácido Pan-
toténico? Beneficios y propiedades | NutriTienda.* Nutritienda. http
s://blog.nutritienda.com/acido-pantotenico/

Petre, A. (2020, June 3). *What is caffeine, and is it good or bad for
health?* Healthline. https://www.healthline.com/nutrition/what-is
-caffeine#metabolism-fat-burning

Podlipnik, S. (2021, January 24). *¿Cómo quitar las manchas en la
cara por un dermatólogo experto?* Dr. Sebastian Podlipnik. https://
www.sebastianpodlipnik.com/quitar-manchas-en-la-cara/

Pond's. (n.d.). *Tipos de manchas que pueden aparecer en tu rostro.* Pond's.   Retrieved   June   11,   2022,   from https://www.ponds.com.ar/articulos/conoce-tu-piel/tono-uniform e/tipos-de-manchas-que-pueden-aparecer-en-tu-rostro.html#:~:text =Las%20cuatro%20categor%C3%ADas%20principales%20son

Press, E. (2018, August 26). *9 consejos para evitar las marcas del acné.* InfoSalus. https://www.infosalus.com/estetica/noticia-consej os-evitar-marcas-acne-20180826081432.html

Ramos-e-Silva, M., Ramos-e-Silva, S., & Carneiro, S. (2015). Acne in women. *British Journal of Dermatology*, *172*, 20–26. https://doi.or g/10.1111/bjd.13638

Rivera, R., & Guerra, A. (2009). Manejo del acné en mujeres mayores de 25 años. *Actas Dermo-Sifiliográficas*, *100*(1), 33–37. https://doi .org/10.1016/S0001-7310(09)70054-7

Robledo, P. L. (2021, November 3). *Si eres latina, tienes que tener más cuidado con las manchas de tu piel.* Cosmopoli- tan. https://www.cosmopolitan.com/es/belleza/tratamientos-cara -cuerpo/a38023701/manchas-piel-latina/#

Rodriguez, E. M. (2017, June 20). *La estructura y funciones de la piel - Blog de CIM Formación.* CIM Grupo de Forma- ción. https://www.cimformacion.com/blog/estetica-y-belleza/capa s-de-la-piel-y-funciones/

Saldana, D. (2021, September 29). *¿Cuáles son los mejores probióti- cos para la piel?* Noticias Sobre Discapacidad, Turismo, Sociedad Y

Economía. https://www.tododisca.com/cuales-son-los-probioticos
-piel/

Saludalia. (n.d.). *La importancia de limpiar la cara a diario*. Saluda
lia.com. https://www.saludalia.com/salud-de-la-piel/la-importanci
a-de-limpiar-la-cara-a-diario

Sanchez, B. C. (2019, December 31). *Por qué TENGO ACNÉ a los
30   AÑOS   y   Cómo   eliminarlo*.   UnCOMO.
https://www.mundodeportivo.com/uncomo/belleza/articulo/por
-que-tengo-acne-a-los-30-anos-y-como-eliminarlo-50087.html

Sanchez-Monge, M. (2019, May 21). *Propiedades y beneficios del se-
lenio*. CuidatePlus. https://cuidateplus.marca.com/alimentacion/n
utricion/2019/05/21/propiedades-beneficios-selenio-170145.html

Santoyo, S. (2019, June 10). *Cremas nutritivas: descubre todos sus
beneficios - ¡Siéntete Guapa!* Sentirte Guapa. https://sentirteguapa
.com/cremas-nutritivas-beneficios/

Schafer, T., Nienhaus, A., Vieluf, D., Berger, J., & Ring, J. (2001).
Epidemiology of acne in the general population: the risk of smoking.
British Journal of Dermatology, 145(1), 100–104. https://doi.org/1
0.1046/j.1365-2133.2001.04290.x

Schwabe, L., & Wolf, O. T. (2009). Stress Prompts Habit Behavior
in Humans. *Journal of Neuroscience, 29*(22), 7191–7198. https://d
oi.org/10.1523/jneurosci.0979-09.2009

Scripps. (2013, July 8). *Can sunscreen reverse skin aging?*
Scripps Health. https://www.scripps.org/news_items/4532-how-t
o-slow-down-your-skin-s-aging

Self-reported facial characteristics associated with aging in a diverse sample of men and women from a multinational Web-based panel survey. (2015). *Journal of the American Academy of Dermatology, 72*(5), AB25. https://doi.org/10.1016/j.jaad.2015.02.112

Sendagorta Cudós, E., & de Lucas Laguna, R. (2009). Tratamiento de la dermatitis atópica. *Pediatría Atención Primaria, 11*, 49–67. https://scielo.isciii.es/scielo.php?script=sci_arttext&pid=S1139-76322009000300004

Sherry, M. (2022, May 3). *Estas son las 10 claves para prevenir el acné adulto.* Estetic. https://www.consalud.es/estetic/bienestar/10-claves-prevenir-acne-adulto_110338_102.html

Sinrich, J. (2018, June 20). *How your skin changes in your 30s—and what you can do about it.* SELF. https://www.self.com/story/skin-care-routine-30s#:~:text=%E2%80%9CCell%20turnover%20slows%20down%2C%20skin

Skin Cancer Foundation. (2018, December 28). *Protector solar: Acerca del protector solar.* La Fundación de Cáncer de Piel. https://cancerdepiel.org/prevencion/proteccion-solar/protector-solar-acerca-del-protector-solar

Streit, L. (2021, June 9). *Omega-3 and acne: What's the connection?* Healthline. https://www.healthline.com/nutrition/omega-3-for-acne

TechnoReviews. (2019, October 21). *Bálsamo labial: aprende a elegir lo mejor de 2020.* TecnoReviews. https://tecnoreviews.online/balsamo-labial/

Vanitatis, C. (2018, November 13). *Qué propiedades tiene la vitamina K y por qué la necesitamos.* Vanitatis.elconfidencial.com . https://www.vanitatis.elconfidencial.com/estilo/belleza/2018-11 -13/que-es-la-vitamina-k_1637821/

Vincent, M. (2014, September 18). *Cómo elegir una crema para piel grasa - 6 pasos.* Www.mundodeportivo.com/Uncomo . https://www.mundodeportivo.com/uncomo/belleza/articulo/co mo-elegir-una-crema-para-piel-grasa-29668.html

WebMD. (n.d.). *Top foods high in Vitamin E.* WebMD. https://ww w.webmd.com/diet/foods-high-in-vitamin-e#1

WHO. (n.d.). *Vitamin A deficiency.* World Health Organization. https://www.who.int/data/nutrition/nlis/info/vitamin-a-defi ciency#:~:text=Deficiency%20of%20vitamin%20A%20is

Women's Health. (2016, December 15). *Todo lo que el magnesio puede hacer por tu piel.* Women's Health. https://www.womenshe althmag.com/es/salud-bienestar/a2001329/magnesio-beneficios/

World Health Organization. (n.d.). *Radiation: The ultraviolet (UV) index.* World Health Organization. https://www.who.int/news-roo m/questions-and-answers/item/radiation-the-ultraviolet-(uv)-index

Zonadamas. (2021, June 23). *Crema para piel seca: ¿Cuál es la mejor del 2022?* ZONADAMAS. https://www.zonadamas.mx/crema-pa ra-piel-seca/

Image References

Andréa. D. (2020). *Melancholic ethnic woman with makeup and curly hair near mirror.* Pexels. https://www.pexels.com/photo/melancholic-ethnic-woman-with-makeup-and-curly-hair-near-mirror-4289680/

Cottonbro. (2021). *Woman putting face cream on cheek.* Pexels.

Cottonbro. (2020). *Woman lying on blue textile.* Pexels. https://www.pexels.com/photo/woman-lying-on-blue-textile-3997993/

Lach, R. (2021). *Person holding a dropper with liquid.* Pexels. https://www.pexels.com/photo/person-holding-a-dropper-with-liquid-8140908/

Monstera. (2021). *Anonymous black woman with clay mask.* Pexels.

Pixabay. (2017). *Spilled bottle of yellow capsule pills.* Pexels. https://www.pexels.com/photo/spilled-bottle-of-yellow-capsule-pills-208518/

Santos, V. (2019). *Woman washing her face with water.* Pexels.https://www.pexels.com/photo/woman-washing-her-face-with-water-2087954/

Shvets, A. (2020). *Person in white long sleeve shirt holding gray and yellow tube.* Pexels. https://www.pexels.com/photo/people-woman-hand-industry-4586856/

Shvets, A. (2020). *Crop person with smear of face cream.* Pexels. https://www.pexels.com/photo/crop-person-with-smear-of-face-cream-5217926/

Tarazevich, A. (2020). *Woman with white towel on head scrubbing her face*. Pexels.

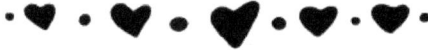

· ♥ · ♥ · ♥ · ♥ · ♥ ·

www.artemixbeauty.com

www.ingramcontent.com/pod-product-compliance
Lightning Source LLC
Chambersburg PA
CBHW052113030426
42335CB00025B/2959